Secrets to staying forever young in your 40s, 50s, and 60s

The science and strategy of thriving in every decade while embracing confidence and grace

Introduction

Let's face it: everyone wants to remain young. We constantly encounter claims of eternal youth, from wrinkle creams to fad diets. Despite all of the marketing tactics, aging is a natural part of life. The question is not whether we can stop aging but how we can age well. And the good news? Scientific evidence shows we have more control over aging than previously thought.

We are approaching a new era in which our lifestyle choices can affect not just how long but also how well we live. Forget quick fixes and so-called "miracle cures." The genuine secret to aging well resides in our daily choices—what we eat, how we move, and even how we think. Scientific advancements have provided us with the keys to living not only longer but also fuller, more vibrant lives. While time cannot be reversed, the symptoms of aging—disease, physical deterioration, and mental fog—can be delayed and, in many cases, averted.

This book will walk you through the science-based strategies. It will teach you how to eat for life, move to build your body, and adopt mindsets that keep you resilient. Everything in this book is based on data and research, and it is intended to provide you with effective strategies to naturally delay the aging process while avoiding fads and myths.

Unlike the bogus claims of anti-aging products, our method is unique. There are no quick cures here, simply realistic, scientifically established solutions that you may apply in your daily life. Whether you're in your 30s, 50s, or older, the techniques in this book will help you regain control of your health, increase your vitality, and add years to your life. Aging is inevitable, but how you age is entirely up to you. Ready to get started? Let's dive in.

Chapter One

Understanding the Aging Process

Aging is one of the few universal experiences we all have. It's unavoidable, yet how each person perceives it varies greatly. Some people appear to remain spry and sharp well into their golden years, whereas others begin to fade in their 40s or 50s. Why is that? The answer is a complicated blend of biology and lifestyle, and understanding what happens at the molecular level is the first step toward gaining control over how we age.

Science of Biological Aging

Aging is fundamentally a biological process that occurs in every cell in our bodies. As we age, our cells begin to amass damage, lose their ability to repair themselves, and eventually cease to function entirely. This cellular aging process is driven by a number of fundamental elements, each of which has a distinct impact on how our bodies develop over time.

Telomere shortening is one of the best-known culprits. Telomeres are protective caps at the ends of our chromosomes, similar to the plastic tips on shoelaces that keep them from fraying. Each time a cell divides, its telomeres become somewhat shorter. As the telomeres shorten over time, the cell's ability to divide properly is compromised, resulting in cellular aging and, finally, cell death. In summary, telomeres function as biological clocks, counting down the number of times our cells may regenerate.

Another important factor is **cellular senescence**. As cells age and collect damage, they enter a state known as senescence. These senescent cells no longer function correctly, and they produce inflammatory molecules that can harm nearby healthy cells. This process leads to tissue and organ aging, resulting in both visible and hidden indications of age, such as wrinkles and cognitive deterioration.

However, there is more to aging than telomeres and senescence. Other factors, such as **oxidative stress**, also come into play. Throughout our lives, our cells are constantly exposed to dangerous chemicals known as free radicals. These molecules are byproducts of regular metabolic activities, but they may also be caused by external influences such as pollution or radiation. Free radicals cause damage to our cells, which accumulates over time, contributing to aging and age-related disorders.

Finally, there's **mitochondrial malfunction**, which is frequently considered a sign of aging. Mitochondria, the powerhouses of our cells, generate the energy we require to function. As humans age, mitochondria become less efficient, producing less energy and emitting more toxic byproducts such as free radicals. This loss in mitochondrial activity adds to muscle weakness, fatigue, and the general slowing that is associated with aging.

Why Do Some People Age Better Than Others

If aging is a universal process, why do some people appear to age more gracefully than others? This is where the age-old dispute between **genetics** and **lifestyle** comes into play. It's true that genetics influence how we age. Some people are just born with genes that protect them against age-related ailments or allow them to look young for longer periods of time. However, as powerful as genetics are, they are only one piece of the puzzle. In fact, **lifestyle decisions** frequently play a larger role in shaping how we age.

Consider telomere shortening, for instance. While everyone's telomeres shrink as they age, evidence indicates that lifestyle factors such as nutrition, exercise, and stress management might influence how quickly this happens. According to research, persons who eat a diet rich in whole, plant-based foods, exercise regularly, and practice stress-reduction techniques such as mindfulness or meditation had longer telomeres than those who live a more sedentary, processed-food-filled lifestyle.

Similarly, oxidative stress can be influenced by our diet and lifestyle. Fruits and vegetables include antioxidants, which help neutralize free radicals and reduce the damage they can do to our cells. Exercise is also significant in this situation. While exercise momentarily increases the creation of free radicals, it also strengthens the body's natural antioxidant defenses, resulting in a long-term favorable benefit.

Let's not forget about **sleep**, one of the most neglected aspects of healthy aging. Deep sleep allows our bodies to repair damaged cells, eliminate poisons, and even repair DNA damage. Chronic sleep deprivation, on the other hand, accelerates cellular aging and raises the risk of a variety of disorders, including heart disease and Alzheimer's.

Social relationships play an unexpectedly major function in aging. According to studies, those with strong social relationships live longer and healthier lives than those who are socially isolated. A sense of community, purpose, and connection with others can reduce stress, improve mental health, and even promote physical health. The world's longest-lived populations, such as Okinawa, Japan, and Sardinia, Italy, are noted not only for their healthy diets but also for their strong social bonds and sense of purpose, known as "ikigai" or "reason for being."

Aging is inevitable, yet how we age is largely under our control.

It's straightforward to conceive of aging as an uncontrollable natural process. However, as science continues to unravel the mysteries of aging, it becomes obvious that humans have more control over the process than previously imagined. While we can't modify our genetic code or stop time from moving forward, we can make choices that delay the biological clock.

By eating the correct foods, being active, getting adequate rest, and creating meaningful social interactions, we can protect our cells from harm, keep our mitochondria operating smoothly, and even alter the length of our telomeres. Aging may be unavoidable, but how we age—whether we thrive or simply survive—is determined by the decisions we make on a daily basis.

In the following chapters, we'll go deeper into each of these lifestyle factors, giving you the science-backed techniques you need to live a longer, healthier, and more vibrant life. We cannot stop the clock, but we can surely slow it down.

Chapter 2

The Science Behind Anti-Aging Foods

What we consume impacts all of our cells at their very core, from our DNA to the mitochondria that power our bodies. When it comes to anti-aging, food can be an extremely effective strategy. While there is no magic pill, decades of studies have demonstrated that entire, plant-based diets, such as the Mediterranean and anti-inflammatory diets, can play an important role in slowing down the aging process on the cellular level.

How plant-based diets protect cells

At the heart of aging is **oxidative stress**, a condition created by an imbalance between free radicals—unstable chemicals that can harm cells—and the body's ability to neutralize them with antioxidants. Free radicals are naturally formed throughout metabolism, but environmental conditions such as pollution, smoking, and a poor diet can boost their production. Free radical damage eventually causes cellular aging, inflammation, and chronic diseases, such as heart disease, cancer, and diabetes.

This is where complete, plant-based diets come into play. They are high in **antioxidants,** which are chemicals that neutralize free radicals and keep them from causing damage. What is the best part? These diets do more than only provide antioxidants to the body; they also aid in lowering inflammation, which is another major cause of aging and disease.

Consider the **Mediterranean diet**, which is widely regarded as one of the world's healthiest eating habits. It focuses on fruits, vegetables, whole grains, legumes, nuts, seeds, and olive oil, with moderate amounts of fish and poultry and little red meat and sugar. This diet is high in **polyphenols, carotenoids, flavonoids, and vitamins C and E**, all of which serve as antioxidants. Polyphenols, such as those present in olive oil and red wine, have been demonstrated to lower oxidative stress and inflammation, reducing cellular aging.

But what distinguishes the Mediterranean diet is its potential to lower chronic, low-grade inflammation, sometimes known as **"inflammaging**." This form of inflammation is a major cause of age-related disorders such as Alzheimer's, heart disease, and cancer. The diet's high quantities of **omega-3 fatty acids**, found in fish such as salmon and flaxseeds, offer powerful anti-inflammatory capabilities, protecting cells from harm and lowering the risk of chronic disease.

The power of Anti-Inflammatory Foods

The anti-inflammatory diet is closely related to the Mediterranean diet, as it focuses on foods that help reduce inflammation throughout the body. Inflammation is the body's natural defense mechanism, but when it becomes chronic, it hastens aging and raises the risk of illness. The anti-inflammatory diet includes many of the same foods as the Mediterranean diet, but it focuses more on foods that have anti-inflammatory qualities.

Berries, such as blueberries, strawberries, and raspberries, are high in **anthocyanins**, potent antioxidants that have been demonstrated to lower inflammation indicators in the body. According to studies, persons who eat berries on a regular basis had reduced levels of inflammatory markers such as C-reactive protein, which are linked to aging and chronic disease.

Turmeric, a spice commonly used in Indian cuisine, is another prominent anti-aging ingredient. Turmeric's main ingredient, **curcumin**, has been demonstrated to have powerful anti-inflammatory and antioxidant properties. Curcumin has been shown in multiple trials to reduce inflammation at the cellular level, and it is also being studied for its ability to protect against neurodegenerative disorders such as Alzheimer's, which are caused by chronic inflammation.

Gut health: the microbiome's role in aging.

One of the most intriguing recent discoveries is the link between nutrition, intestinal health, and aging. Human gut's billions of bacteria, known as the **microbiome**, are crucial to human health. As we become older, the variety of our microbiome decreases, and an imbalance of gut bacteria has been linked to chronic diseases, inflammation, and even shorter lifespans.

A diet rich in whole, plant-based foods supports a healthy microbiome by supplying **prebiotics**, which are fibers that feed beneficial gut bacteria. Foods high in prebiotics include onions, garlic, bananas, and asparagus, which help to maintain a diverse and healthy microbiota. Diets high in processed foods, sugar, and unhealthy fats, on the other hand, can result in an excess of harmful bacteria, which contributes to inflammation and accelerates aging.

Take fermented foods like yogurt, sauerkraut, and kimchi as an example. These foods include **probiotics**, which are beneficial bacteria that help keep the gut healthy. According to research, persons who eat fermented foods on a daily basis have improved gut health and lower levels of inflammation, which may contribute to aging more slowly.

Specific Nutrients' Anti-Aging Effects

While entire meals are more beneficial than isolated nutrients, several vitamins and minerals have received substantial research for their anti-aging benefits.

- **Vitamin C**, found in citrus fruits, bell peppers, and leafy greens, is a potent antioxidant that helps protect skin cells from oxidative stress and supports collagen production, which keeps skin firm and youthful

- **Vitamin E**, found in nuts, seeds, and spinach, works with Vitamin C to protect cells from oxidative damage.

- **Omega-3 fatty acids**, found in fatty fish, flaxseeds, and chia seeds, offer anti-inflammatory qualities and protect against cardiovascular disease, which is more common as we age.

- **Resveratrol**, a polyphenol found in red grapes and berries, activates genes linked to lifespan and may have anti-aging effects on the cardiovascular system and brain.

Real-life examples of anti-aging diets in action

The lifespan of populations in **Blue Zones**, areas where people live substantially longer than average, demonstrates the effectiveness of plant-based diets in reducing the aging process. People in Okinawa, Japan, and Ikaria, Greece, live into their 90s and beyond, thanks in large part to their diets. These communities eat mostly plant-based foods, including vegetables, beans, and whole grains, with very little meat or processed goods. Their diets are high in antioxidants, anti-inflammatory chemicals, and fiber, all of which help protect their cells and contribute to their amazing longevity.

For example, the Okinawan diet is high in **sweet potatoes**, which contain beta-carotene, a potent antioxidant that protects the skin and cells from oxidative stress. They also eat a lot of **seaweed**, which contains anti-aging chemicals, including fucoidan, a polysaccharide that has been demonstrated to improve immunological function and cellular repair.

Building an Anti-Aging Diet

The foods we eat have a significant impact on how we age, down to the cellular level. We may dramatically slow down the aging process and protect ourselves from age-related diseases by eating a full, plant-based diet rich in antioxidants, anti-inflammatory chemicals, and minerals that promote cellular health. The goal is to consume a wide variety of fruits and vegetables, incorporate healthy fats, and limit processed foods and added sugars.

Remember, aging is unavoidable, but by making wise eating choices, we may manage how gracefully we age.

Every bite counts. The evidence is clear: whole, plant-based foods are more than simply fuel for our bodies; they are medicine, protecting our cells, supporting our microbiome, and promoting our well-being at any age.

Top anti-aging nutrients for longevity and cellular health

The aging process may be unavoidable, but the rate at which it occurs can be altered by the nutrients we ingest. The correct vitamins, antioxidants, and other bioactive molecules can help protect our cells, decrease the aging process, and lower the risk of age-related disorders. Let's look at the most powerful anti-aging nutrients—vitamins, antioxidants, omega-3s, polyphenols, and more—and how they can help us age better.

1. Vitamin C: The Skin Protector.

Vitamin C is a most potent **antioxidant** that plays an important role in skin health and longevity. As an antioxidant, it protects cells from oxidative stress generated by free radicals, which can hasten aging. Free radicals are unstable chemicals that harm cells, proteins, and DNA, causing apparent indications of aging like wrinkles as well as more serious problems like heart disease or cancer.

Vitamin C is also essential for **collagen formation**, which maintains skin that is tight and robust. As we age, collagen production naturally slows, resulting in drooping skin and wrinkles. Consuming vitamin C-rich foods—such as citrus fruits, bell peppers, broccoli, and strawberries—can help the body generate collagen, keeping the skin youthful and supple.

For example, research has shown that those who consume more Vitamin C have fewer wrinkles and have less age-related dryness. What's the reason? Vitamin C not only protects the skin from external stressors like pollution, but it also boosts the body's ability to heal damaged skin cells.

2. Vitamin E—the Cellular Shield

Vitamin E and Vitamin C work together to protect cells from oxidative damage. It's especially crucial for skin health because it protects against UV radiation and other environmental stressors.

This fat-soluble vitamin is abundant in the skin's outer layer, where it serves as a barrier against moisture loss and injury. It is a powerful antioxidant, similar to Vitamin C that neutralizes free radicals and prevents cellular aging.

Vitamin E-rich foods include almonds and hazelnuts, seeds (such as sunflower seeds), spinach, and avocados. A diet high in Vitamin E can help with smoother skin, fewer fine wrinkles, and stronger cell membranes, making it an essential component of any anti-aging diet.

3. Omega-3 Fatty Acids: The Inflammatory Fighter

Chronic inflammation, often known as "inflammaging," is one of the most well-studied causes of aging. This low-level, long-term inflammation contributes to age-related disorders such as arthritis, cardiovascular problems, and even cognitive impairment. Omega-3 fatty acids are widely recognized for their potent **anti-inflammatory properties.**

Omega-3s, notably **EPA** (eicosapentaenoic acid) and **DHA** (docosahexaenoic acid), found in fatty fish such as salmon, mackerel, and sardines, aid in reducing inflammation all over the body. They are also beneficial to brain health, protecting against neurodegenerative illnesses such as Alzheimer's. According to studies, those who consume more Omega-3 fatty acids experience slower rates of cognitive deterioration as they age.

Omega-3s also improve **heart health** by lowering blood triglyceride levels, blood pressure, and the risk of arrhythmias. Omega-3s can help keep your heart healthy as you age by reducing inflammation, which is a key cause of heart disease.

For vegetarians and vegans, plant-based Omega-3 sources include **ALA** (alpha-linolenic acid), which can be found in flaxseeds, chia seeds, and walnuts. While ALA is less powerful than EPA and DHA, it nevertheless has protective effects and can be transformed in tiny amounts to more accessible forms.

4. Polyphenols: The Longevity Compounds.

Polyphenols are plant-based chemicals with strong antioxidant and anti-inflammatory properties, making them important players in the battle against aging. Polyphenols, which can be found in a wide range of fruits, vegetables, herbs, spices, and beverages such as green tea and red wine, have been widely researched for their role in prolonging longevity and lowering the risk of chronic diseases.

Resveratrol, a well-known polyphenol, can be found in the skins of red grapes and berries, as well as red wine. Resveratrol has been demonstrated to activate genes associated with longevity, specifically those involved in cellular repair and protection. This polyphenol also mimics the effects of caloric restriction, which has been associated with a longer lifespan and lower risk of age-related diseases in various animal studies.

Other polyphenols, such as **flavonoids** (found in berries, citrus fruits, and onions) and **catechins** (rich in green tea), help to reduce oxidative stress and inflammation and protect the brain against age-related cognitive decline. Regular consumption of polyphenol-rich foods has been related to improved heart health, sharper cognitive performance, and even longer lifespans in societies with high polyphenol diets.

5. Coenzyme Q10 (CoQ10), the Cellular Energizer.

As we age, the effectiveness of our cells' mitochondria—often referred to as the cell's "powerhouses"—declines. This decline in mitochondrial activity reduces energy levels and contributes to age-related weariness and muscular weakening. **CoenzymeQ10 (CoQ10)** is a molecule that helps mitochondria generate energy, and its levels normally decline as we age.

CoQ10 is also an antioxidant, which protects cells from oxidative damage and helps keep skin elastic. Supplementation with CoQ10 has been demonstrated to increase mitochondrial activity and reduce fatigue in older persons. CoQ10 also promotes heart health by lowering oxidative stress and boosting blood flow, making it a critical component for preserving vitality as we age.

Foods such as fatty fish (salmon and tuna), organ meats, and whole grains include trace amounts of CoQ10, although supplementation may be required for optimal levels, particularly in older persons.

6. Vitamin D: A Bone and Immunity Supporter

Vitamin D is essential not only for **bone health** as we age but also to strengthen the immune system. As we age, the body's ability to produce vitamin D from sunshine decreases, thereby increasing the risk of osteoporosis, fractures, and immunological dysfunction.

According to research, vitamin D reduces inflammation, protects against chronic diseases, such as heart disease and cancer, and promotes brain function. Adequate vitamin D levels have been related to improved cognitive function, but deficiencies have been connected to an increased risk of dementia and Alzheimer's disease.

Natural sources of vitamin D include fatty fish (such as salmon and mackerel), egg yolks, and fortified foods like milk and orange juice. However, due to the difficulties of receiving enough Vitamin D through diet alone, supplementation is frequently recommended, particularly for older persons.

A Nutrient-Rich Approach to Aging Well

The aging process cannot be stopped, but with the correct nutrition, we may certainly slow it down and stay healthy. We can protect our cells, support our mitochondria, and lower our risk of chronic diseases by eating a nutrient-dense, plant-based diet rich in

antioxidants, anti-inflammatory compounds, and important vitamins.

The key to aging properly is not in miracle drugs or gimmicks but in the meals we consume every day. From Vitamin C's skin-saving properties to Omega-3s' anti-inflammatory power and polyphenols' longevity-boosting benefits, these nutrients work together to promote a long, healthy life.

Chapter3

Meal Planning for Youthful Living.

When it comes to aging gracefully, the ancient saying, "You are what you eat," has never been more accurate. Foods we eat have a significant impact on cellular health, inflammation, and the body's ability to repair and regenerate. Proper meal planning, with a focus on anti-aging nutrients, can help you slow the aging process, improve cognitive and physical function, and lower your risk of age-related disorders. Here, we'll look at how to include these nutrients in healthy, enjoyable meals that promote youthfulness.

- **Breakfast: An energizing and anti-inflammatory start.**

Meal: Blueberry Chia Pudding with Walnuts

This dish incorporates numerous powerful anti-aging ingredients. **Blueberries** are packed with **anthocyanins,** which lower inflammation and protect the brain from oxidative stress. **Chia seeds** are high **in omega-3 fatty acids**, which lower inflammation and promote heart health; **walnuts** contain additional omega-3s and beneficial fats.

Recipe

• Add two tablespoons of chia seeds.

• 1/2 cup unsweetened almond milk.

• 1/2 cup fresh blueberries.

• 1 tablespoon crumbled walnuts

• 1 tsp honey (optional)

• Add ½ teaspoon vanilla extract.

Combine the chia seeds, almond milk, and vanilla essence. Let it sit in the refrigerator overnight to thicken. In the morning, top with blueberries, walnuts, and honey, if preferred. This breakfast is high in **fiber**, which keeps you full and promotes digestive health, and the antioxidants and omega-3s protect your cells from aging.

Why it works: Blueberries have been demonstrated to increase cognitive function and lower the risk of Alzheimer's disease, making them an ideal breakfast food. Chia seeds provide long-lasting energy, and the omega-3s in both chia and walnuts combat chronic inflammation, which is a major factor in aging.

- **Mid-Morning Snack: Increase Your Antioxidants**.

Meal: Green tea with a handful of almonds

Green tea contains a high concentration of **catechins**, a type of polyphenol with powerful antioxidant properties. It has been demonstrated to benefit cognitive function, improve cardiovascular health, and lower the risk of cancer. This snack, which includes **vitamin E-rich almonds**, promotes skin health and protects cells from oxidative damage.

Why it works: Regular green tea consumption has been related to higher life expectancy, notably among Asian communities such as those in Japan's Okinawa region. Almonds help preserve youthful skin by eliminating free radicals, a major cause of aging.

Lunch: A Mediterranean Powerhouse.

Meal: Quinoa Salad with Spinach, Avocado, and Olive Oil

The Mediterranean diet is a recognized anti-aging powerhouse, and this meal is high in key nutrients. **Quinoa** is a complete protein that contains all nine essential amino acids, which aid in muscle maintenance as we age. **Spinach** contains high levels of **vitamin C** and **vitamin A**, all of which are essential for keeping youthful skin and health. **Avocados** are high in **healthy fats** and **potassium**, which help prevent inflammation and maintain heart health. **Olive oil**, rich in **polyphenols**, protects against oxidative stress and chronic inflammation.

Recipe

- One cup cooked quinoa.

- One handful of fresh spinach.

- ½ sliced avocado

- Add 2 tablespoons of extra virgin olive oil.

- Add 1 tablespoon lemon juice.

- Add salt and pepper to taste.

- Sprinkle sunflower seeds for crunch.

Combine the spinach and avocado with the cooked quinoa. Drizzle olive oil and lemon juice over the salad, then season with salt, pepper, and sunflower seeds for extra vitamin E.

Why it works: Quinoa's protein concentration promotes muscle maintenance, whereas spinach contains antioxidants such as lutein, which protect the eyes and skin. Avocados include heart-healthy monounsaturated fats, while olive oil's polyphenols prevent oxidative stress and promote long-term cellular health.

- **Afternoon Snack: Fiber and Omega-3 Boost.**

Meal: Flaxseed and Oat Energy Bites

These energy bites are produced from **flaxseeds**, which contain **ALA (alpha-linolenic acid)**, an omega-3 fatty acid that promotes brain function and decreases inflammation. **Oats** include **beta-glucans,** a form of soluble fiber that reduces cholesterol and promotes intestinal health.

Recipe

• One cup of rolled oats.

• 2 tablespoons ground flaxseed.

• Add 2 tablespoons almond butter.

Add 1 tablespoon of honey.

• Add 1 teaspoon vanilla extract.

• ¼ cup dark chocolate chips (optional).

Combine all of the ingredients, shape little balls, and refrigerate. These bites are quick to make and, thanks to their omega-3 and fiber content, have anti-aging properties.

Why it works: Flaxseeds are one of the richest plant sources of omega-3 fatty acids, which have been linked to lower risk of heart disease and improved cognitive performance. Oats keep you full while also promoting intestinal health, which is critical for long-term well-being.

• **Dinner is anti-inflammatory and nutrient-dense**.

Meal: Grilled salmon with sweet potatoes and broccoli.

Salmon is high in **EPA** and **DHA**, omega-3 fatty acids that benefit the heart and brain. **Sweet potatoes** are high in

beta-carotene, a precursor to vitamin A that is essential for preserving skin suppleness and protecting against UV radiation. **Broccoli** contains a variety of anti-aging properties, including **sulforaphane**, which improves detoxification, and vitamin C, which aids in collagen formation.

Recipe

• One fillet of wild-caught salmon.

• Cut 1 sweet potato into cubes.

• One cup of steamed broccoli.

• Combine olive oil, salt, and pepper for seasoning.

Roast the sweet potatoes with a sprinkle of olive oil at 400°F (200°C) for 30-35 minutes. Grill or bake the salmon until it's cooked through. Serve with steamed broccoli for a nutritious, anti-inflammatory lunch.

Why it works: Omega-3s in salmon reduce inflammation, sweet potatoes improve skin health, and broccoli has detoxifying substances that protect cells from injury. Together, they provide a supper high in nutrients that promote longevity.

- **Evening snack: Skin and Brain Support.**

Meal: Dark chocolate and walnuts

Finish the day with a treat that nevertheless helps safeguard your body. **Dark chocolate** contains **flavonoids**, which promote circulation and cognitive function, and **walnuts** have additional omega-3 fatty acids, which reduce inflammation.

Why it works: Research indicates that eating dark chocolate increases blood flow to the brain, which aids cognitive performance as we age. Walnuts' high antioxidant concentration protects cells from free radical damage.

Conclusion: Strategic Nutritional Planning for Longevity

Incorporating these meals and snacks into your daily routine assures a steady supply of the nutrients that combat aging at the cell level. The goal is to consume a range of full, plant-based foods high in antioxidants, anti-inflammatory chemicals, and important vitamins. Whether you start your day with blueberry chia pudding or end it with a square of dark chocolate and walnuts, these foods work together to promote vibrant health, brain function, skin protection, and a lower risk of age-related disorders.

Chapter4

Action Step: A 7-Day Anti-Aging Meal Plan with a Complete Shopping List.

This 7-day meal plan will guide you through a week of eating to encourage longevity and anti-aging, with an emphasis on nutrient-dense foods high in antioxidants, omega-3 fatty acids, vitamins, and anti-inflammatory chemicals. Each day includes meals meant to promote cellular health, increase skin elasticity, improve cognitive function, and reduce inflammation—all of which are important factors in slowing the aging process.

Day 1

- **Breakfast**: Blueberry Chia Pudding with Walnuts.

- **Snack**: Green tea with almonds.

- **Lunch**: Quinoa salad topped with spinach, avocado, and olive oil.

- **Snack**: flaxseed and oat energy bites.

- **Dinner**: grilled fish with sweet potatoes and steamed broccoli.

- **Snack**: Dark chocolate with walnuts.

Day 2

- **Breakfast**: Oatmeal with berries, flaxseed, and almond butter.

- **Snack**: Apple slices and almond butter.

- **Lunch**: lentil and vegetable soup served with mixed greens.

- **Snack**: Carrot sticks with hummus.

- **Dinner**: Baked cod, roasted Brussels sprouts, and quinoa.

- **Snack**: Dark chocolate.

Day 3

- **Breakfast**: Avocado toast on whole grain bread with a poached egg.

- **Snack**: A handful of mixed nuts (almonds, walnuts, hazelnuts).

- **Lunch**: Mediterranean chickpea salad with olive oil and lemon.

- **Snack**: Sliced cucumber with tzatziki.

- **Dinner**: Stir-fried tofu, veggies, and brown rice.

- **Snack**: Greek yogurt topped with flaxseeds and honey.

Day 4

- **Breakfast**: Smoothie with spinach, banana, almond butter, and chia seeds.

- **Snack**: A modest amount of sunflower seeds.

- **Lunch**: Spinach and kale salad with grilled chicken, olive oil, and feta cheese.

- **Snack**: mixed berries.

- **Dinner**: zucchini noodles with tomato sauce, olive oil, and lentil meatballs.

• **Snack**: dark chocolate and walnuts.

Day 5

• **Breakfast**: scrambled eggs with spinach, mushrooms, and avocado.

• **Snack**: Green tea with pumpkin seeds.

• **Lunch**: Sweet potato and black bean tacos topped with avocado.

• **Snack**: Apple slices and a spoonful of peanut butter.

• **Dinner**: Grilled chicken, roasted carrots, and quinoa

• **Snack**: A small bowl of mixed berries with a spoonful of Greek yogurt

Day 6

• **Breakfast**: Whole grain bread with almond butter and sliced bananas.

• **Snack**: raw almonds.

- **Lunch**: Grilled vegetable wrap, hummus, and mixed greens.

- **Snack**: Small handful of walnuts.

- **Dinner**: Baked fish with wild rice and steamed asparagus.

- **Snack**: Dark chocolate and green tea.

Day 7

- **Breakfast**: Chia seed pudding topped with blueberries and honey.

- **Snack**: Carrot sticks with hummus.

- **Lunch**: Quinoa bowl with kale, chickpeas, and tahini dressing.

- **Snack**: Small handful of mixed nuts.

- **Dinner**: Lentil soup and mixed greens salad.

- **Snack**: Dark chocolate with a tiny glass of red wine.

Complete shopping list for 7 days

Fruits

• Blueberries, fresh or frozen

• Mixed berries (strawberries, raspberries, and blackberries)

• Bananas

• Apples

• Avocados

• Lemons

Vegetables

• Spinach

• Kale

• Broccoli

• Zucchini

• Brussels sprouts

- Sweet potatoes

- Carrots

- Cucumbers

- Mushrooms

- Asparagus

- Tomatoes for sauce

- Bell peppers

- Mixed greens for salads

- Tofu for stir-fry.

Proteins

- Wild-caught salmon

- Baked cod

- Organic chicken breast (free-range)

- Eggs

- Lentils (dried or canned)

- Chickpeas (dried or canned)

- Black beans (canned)

- Greek yogurt (simple and unsweetened)

- Almond butter

- Peanut butter (unsweetened)

Grain and Seed

- Quinoa

- Brown rice

- Wild rice

- Whole grain bread

- Oatmeal (rolling or steel-cut)

- Chia Seeds

- Flaxseeds

- Sunflower seeds

- Pumpkin seeds

Nuts

• Walnuts

• Almonds

• Hazelnuts

• Mixed nuts

Dairy (or dairy alternatives)

• Feta cheese

• Unsweetened almond milk

• Cold-pressed and extra virgin olive oil

Spices and seasonings

• Olive Oil

• Tahini (salad dressing)

• Green Tea.

• Dark chocolate (70% cacao or more)

• Honey.

• Red wine (in moderation).

Breaking It Down: Why These Choices Matter

Fruits and Vegetables: This plan focuses on nutrient-dense, colorful fruits and vegetables to ensure a high intake of antioxidants, polyphenols, and vitamins C and E, which protect against oxidative stress and inflammation.

Omega-3s: Salmon, walnuts, and chia seeds are high in omega-3 fatty acids, which help battle chronic inflammation, a significant cause of aging and disease.

Protein Sources: Plant-based proteins like lentils and chickpeas, as well as lean animal proteins like chicken and fish, aid in preserving muscle mass and lowering the risk of sarcopenia (age-related muscle loss).

Fiber-rich carbs: Quinoa, oats, and brown rice provide complex carbs and fiber that not only enhance intestinal health but also assist in maintaining stable blood sugar levels, which is essential for long-term metabolic health.

Healthy Fats: Avocados, olive oil, and almonds include heart-healthy monounsaturated fats that promote brain function and protect skin from damage.

Dark chocolate and green tea: These two additives pack a significant antioxidant punch. Dark chocolate contains flavonoids, which boost circulation and cognitive function, whereas green tea catechins lower inflammation and increase longevity.

A Sustainable Path to Youthful Living

This meal plan focuses on nutrient-dense, complete foods that have been found to lower inflammation, improve heart and brain health, and increase longevity. By following these recipes and stocking your kitchen with the goods suggested, you may take practical steps toward aging gracefully—without resorting to rigid diets or quick solutions.

Chapter 5

Exercise and Movement for Life.

Why Movement Matters

Movement may be the best ally for decreasing the aging process. Regular physical exercise not only preserves **muscle mass** and **bone density** but also ensures that your **cardiovascular system** functions properly. As we age, the body naturally loses muscle mass known as **sarcopenia** and bone density, increasing the risk of fractures and osteoporosis. But there's positive news: physical activity can considerably slow down these processes, allowing you to keep strength, flexibility, and endurance far into your golden years. Let's look at the facts behind why activity is essential for a long and healthy life.

Muscle Mass and Sarcopenia: Using or Losing It

Muscle loss is a major factor in the physical decline associated with aging. If you don't actively try to preserve your muscle mass, it can drop by 3–5% per decade, beginning in your 30s. Without regular exercise, you could lose up to 30% of your muscular mass by the age of 70. This process, called **sarcopenia**,can cause decreased mobility, balance difficulties, and an increased risk of falls and injury.

Resistance exercise is one of the most effective techniques to reverse natural muscle atrophy. Resistance training, whether done with weights, resistance bands, or bodyweight exercises such as squats and push-ups, promotes **muscle hypertrophy**, or growth. When you engage your muscles regularly, they adapt by becoming stronger and larger to match the demands placed on them. This not only helps to preserve mobility and strength, but it also improves **metabolic health** because muscular tissue burns more calories than fat.

In one study, older adults who participated in resistance training for only 16 weeks saw a 30% gain in muscle strength, demonstrating that it is never too late to begin exercising and seeing effects.

Tip: Aim for at **least 2-3 sessions of resistance exercise each week**, with emphasis on all major muscle groups. Squats, lunges, and push-ups are terrific exercises for preserving muscle mass and increasing strength as you age.

Bone Density and Osteoporosis: Strengthening the Skeleton

Although you may not notice, your bones weaken with age. **Osteopenia**, the precursor of **osteoporosis**, affects a large proportion of the elderly population, particularly women after menopause. When osteoporosis develops, bones become brittle and more prone to fractures, significantly reducing quality of life.

This is where movement comes in. Weight-bearing exercises like walking, running, and even dancing put stress on your bones. This stress causes your body to deposit additional minerals into your bones, including **calcium** and **phosphorus**, which enhance their density and strength. Activities that require your body to work against gravity, such as **hiking** or **resistance training**, are especially effective at maintaining bone mass.

For example, research has shown that frequent weight-bearing exercises can lower the incidence of hip fractures by up to 40%.

Tip: Add at least 30 minutes of weight-bearing movement to your daily regimen. A simple activity such as **brisk walking** can help preserve bone density, and mixing it with resistance training provides an additional boost to skeletal strength. Cardiovascular health: keep the heart pumping.

The heart, like any other muscle, requires regular exercise to maintain its strength. Cardiovascular activity, often known as **aerobic exercise**, is essential for keeping our hearts healthy as we age. It keeps your blood arteries flexible, lowers blood pressure, and lowers your chances of getting **heart disease**, the world's leading cause of death.

Regular aerobic activity strengthens the heart, allowing it to pump blood more effectively throughout the body. This increases the flow of **oxygen** and **nutrients** to your tissues, which promotes cellular health and longevity. According to research, **cardiorespiratory fitness** is directly connected with **increased life expectancy** and a lower risk of chronic diseases such as diabetes and hypertension.

For example, in a landmark study, people who engaged in 150 minutes of moderate-intensity aerobic activity per week lowered their risk of cardiovascular disease by 30%.

Tip: Each week, do at least **150 minutes of moderate areobic exercise**, such as brisk walking, cycling, or swimming. If you're short on time, you can choose **75 minutes of rigorous activity,** such as running or high-intensity interval training (HIIT).

Balance, flexibility, and mobility: maintaining agility as you age

It's not simply about developing strength and endurance. To maintain independence and avoid falls as we age, we must also work on our **balance, flexibility, and mobility**. Falls are one of the main causes of injury in older persons, and they can often lead to a series of health issues. **Yoga, Tai Chi,** and **Pilates** are all wonderful kinds of exercise that improve these important aspects of physical fitness.

Balance exercise, like standing on one leg or walking heel-to-toe, can increase your proprioception (your body's perception of its position in space), whereas **flexibility training** helps preserve joint range of motion and keeps you limber. This is crucial for everyday actions such as bending down, reaching aloft, or even getting out of a chair.

For example, a study of elderly persons who practiced **Tai Chi** discovered that they saw a 58% reduction in falls while also improving overall stability and flexibility.

Tip: Incorporate **balance exercises** and **stretching routines** to your weekly plan, aiming for at least **2 to 3 sessions per week**. Even a few minutes of stretching after each activity will help preserve flexibility.

The Power of Consistency: Movement as a Lifetime Practice

The key to obtaining the benefits of exercise as we age is **consistency**. While beginning an exercise routine at any age has advantages, the true magic occurs when movement becomes a part of your everyday life. Exercise should not be considered a quick remedy but rather a **long-term commitment** to health and vitality. Regular physical activity helps regulate essential hormones such as **insulin** and **cortisol**, which play important roles in aging and metabolism.

Moving regularly not only benefits your muscles, bones, and cardiovascular system, but it also improves the health of your **nervous system** and **brain**. Exercise has been demonstrated to boost **neuroplasticity**, the brain's ability to build new neural connections, thus protecting against cognitive decline and diseases such as Alzheimer's.

Tip: Find activities you enjoy, such as dancing, swimming, or hiking, and incorporate them into your normal routine. Consistency, rather than intensity, is the key to remaining youthful via activity.

Movement is the Fountain of Youth.

Movement is unquestionably the foundation of a long, healthy life. Whether you're looking to develop muscle, protect your bones, improve your heart health, or increase your flexibility, regular physical activity is your most reliable way to halt the aging process. By committing to a balanced regimen that includes **resistance training**, **aerobic exercise**, and **flexibility work**, you are investing in a future in which you may live independently, vitally, and resiliently.

Hippocrates once said, "Walking is man's best medicine," but we now know that a combination of walking, strength training, and balancing exercises is the greatest prescription for aging well. Keep moving, and you'll be able to live a vibrant life at any age.

Types of Exercise to Combat Aging

Exercise is an effective tool for combating the consequences of aging, both at the cellular level and in preserving general physical and mental health. You may address the key features of aging by incorporating a variety of movement patterns, including **strength training**, **cardiovascular exercise**, and **flexibility and balance work**. Each of these types of exercise is important for maintaining our quality of life as we age.

- Strength training preserves muscle mass and metabolic health.

Strength training, often known as resistance training, is one of the most effective methods for combating age-related muscle loss. **Sarcopenia**, or the slow loss of muscle mass, begins in our 30s and accelerates with age. If no therapies are implemented, muscle loss might accelerate exponentially by the age of 60. But here's the important point: **muscle mass isn't just about strength—it's about metabolism, balance, and even cognitive health**.

When you engage in strength training exercises like weightlifting, bodyweight movements (squats, lunges, push-ups), or resistance band work, you stimulate **muscle hypertrophy**—the growth of muscle fibers. This process makes your body use more energy, which improves **metabolic health** by increasing the quantity of calories expended during rest. Muscles are metabolically active tissues, which means that the more muscle you have, the better your body manages **blood sugar** and **insulin levels**, both of which are important in the prevention of chronic diseases such as diabetes.

For example, research has shown that older persons who engage in resistance exercise can rebuild muscle mass and strength at the same rate as younger adults. For example, research published in the Journal of Gerontology found that persons over the age of 70 who exercised twice a week for 12 weeks improved their muscle strength by 50%.

Tip: To prevent muscle loss, aim to incorporate **strength training** into your routine at least **two to three times a week**. Squats, deadlifts, and presses are especially beneficial, whether performed with free weights or resistance bands. Work on all main muscle groups, including your legs, back, chest, and core.

Cardio: promoting heart health and longevity.

Aerobic exercise, sometimes known as **cardio**, is vital for maintaining heart and lung function. As we age, our chance of developing cardiovascular disorders such as hypertension, heart attacks, and strokes increases. Regular cardiovascular exercise strengthens the heart muscle, increases **circulation**, **decreases blood pressure**, and **promotes arterial flexibility**. When you exercise, your heart pumps more efficiently, and the increased blood flow delivers oxygen and nutrients to your cells, which promotes overall cellular health.

Cardio and Longevity: In addition to the immediate cardiovascular advantages, regular aerobic exercise has been linked to a **longer life expectancy**. A long-term study published in JAMA (Journal of the American Medical Association) discovered that those who consistently engaged in moderate to strenuous aerobic activity lived substantially longer than those who did not. Cardiovascular fitness has been demonstrated to lower the risk of all-cause death by up to 30%.

A survey of over 122,000 Cleveland Clinic patients revealed that individuals with the highest levels of cardiorespiratory fitness had the biggest survival advantage. Interestingly, the benefits were observed across all age groups, implying that it is never too late to begin reaping the benefits of regular cardiovascular activity.

Tip: For optimal effects, aim for **150 minutes of moderate-intensity aerobic exercise** (such as brisk walking, cycling, or swimming) each week, or **75 minutes of strenuous exercise** (such as running or high-intensity interval training). This can be broken down into reasonable daily sessions; just 30 minutes of brisk walking five days a week will improve heart health and longevity.

Flexibility and Balance: Keeping Mobility and Avoiding Injuries

As we age, our **joints stiffen** and our **range of motion** reduces, increasing the risk of injury and falling. In fact, falls are one of the major causes of injury-related mortality among older persons. Flexibility and balance exercises are frequently disregarded, but they are essential components of any anti-aging workout plan. By improving **joint flexibility** and **stability**, you lower the risk of injury and ensure your ability to execute daily activities independently.

Flexibility: Stretching, yoga, and Pilates can all help you maintain your joint range of motion. Over time, the body loses flexibility, making simple movements such as bending over or reaching aloft more difficult. Regular stretching keeps muscles and tendons supple, improves posture, and relieves stiffness, particularly in tight areas such as the lower back, hips, and shoulders.

Balance: As we age, our **proprioception** (or sense of body position in space) deteriorates, affecting our ability to balance. **Tai Chi**, yoga, and simple balancing drills (such as standing on one leg or walking heel-to-toe) can all help in this situation. Improved balance not only helps avoid falls, but it also improves overall coordination and agility.

For example, research published in the **Journal of Aging and Physical Activity** indicated that older persons who practiced Tai Chi on a daily basis reduced their risk of falls by 55%. Tai Chi's slow, deliberate movements increase proprioception, muscle strength, and flexibility, all of which are important in preventing falls.

Tip: Include **flexibility and balance exercise** in your regimen at least **twice or three times per week**. Even 10–15 minutes of regular stretching or yoga can significantly increase flexibility and minimize joint stiffness. For balance, try exercises like standing on one leg while brushing your teeth or including Tai Chi or yoga into your monthly plan.

Integrating all types for a holistic approach.

While each sort of exercise has its own set of advantages, the ultimate power comes from mixing strength training, cardio, and flexibility exercises into a comprehensive fitness routine. This holistic approach guarantees that all systems—muscular, cardiovascular, and skeletal—are properly cared for, laying the groundwork for healthy aging.

Consider a weekly regimen that consists of two days of resistance training, three days of aerobic activity, and two days of flexibility and balance practice. Diversifying your activities helps you avoid injury and overuse while also making your workouts more engaging and sustainable.

Aging may be unavoidable, but how we age is mainly under our control. A balanced exercise routine that includes strength training, cardiovascular work, and flexibility exercises will help you retain muscle mass, protect your heart, enhance your balance, and stay independent for longer. It's never too late to start, and even minor changes can make a big difference in your general health and well-being.

As the saying goes, "The body in motion stays in motion," and staying active is one of the most effective ways to age gracefully, healthily, and vibrantly.

Chapter 6

Exercise Routine: A Balanced Weekly Plan for Every Fitness Level

A well-rounded weekly exercise plan should address all components of healthy aging, including **strength**, **cardiovascular endurance**, **flexibility**, and **balance**. Whether you're a novice or an advanced fitness enthusiast, this practice is intended to fulfill your body's needs at any stage of life, increasing lifespan and functional independence. By deliberately incorporating several sorts of workouts, you may ensure that your body is resilient and capable of handling daily tasks, regardless of your age.

Importance of Balance in an Exercise Routine

The optimum training plan does not focus solely on one aspect, such as muscle development or endurance improvement. It is about creating a comprehensive strategy that keeps all biological systems in balance. **Strength training** helps to preserve muscle mass, **cardio** improves heart and lung function, while **flexibility and balance** exercises keep joints healthy and prevent falls. Together, these components form a formidable defense against the consequences of aging.

The **7-day exercise plan** below includes a combination of these components. It's meant to be flexible, so whether you're a novice or an experienced user, you can modify the intensity to suit your fitness level.

Day One: Strength Training (Full Body)

On Day 1, we emphasize **strength training** to engage all main muscle groups. This helps to preserve muscular mass, prevent sarcopenia, and promote bone health.

- **Squats (3 sets of 10–12 repetitions)** work the **quadriceps, hamstrings, glutes,** and **core.** If you're more advanced, use dumbbells to enhance resistance.

- **Push-ups (3 sets of 10-15 reps)**: A bodyweight exercise that strengthens the **chest, shoulders,** and **triceps**. If normal push-ups are too difficult, perform them on your knees.

- **Deadlifts (3 sets of 8-10 reps)** strengthen the **hamstrings, glutes, lower back,** and **core.** Beginners can start with light dumbbells, while more skilled users can utilize a barbell.

- **Planks (hold for 30 to 60 seconds, 3 sets)** are a static exercise that strengthens the **core**, including the **abdominals, obliques,** and **lower back.**

Tip: If you are new to strength training, start with lesser weights and progressively increase as your muscles adapt. Instead of lifting heavy, focus on appropriate form to limit the risk of injury and ensure that your muscles are correctly engaged.

Day 2: Cardiovascular Exercise.

Cardio is essential for heart health, increasing lung capacity, and lowering the risk of chronic conditions like hypertension and diabetes. On Day 2, we prioritize aerobic activity.

• **Brisk Walking or Jogging (30-45 minutes)**: Choose between brisk walking and steady jogging based on your fitness level. This activity promotes cardiovascular health by boosting heart rate and lung capacity.

• **Cycling (30 minutes)** is a low-impact cardio option suitable for persons with joint concerns. It works the **quads**, **hamstrings**, and **glutes** while delivering an excellent cardiovascular exercise.

Tip: If walking or jogging becomes boring, try **dance** or **aerobic courses**, which may be both enjoyable and beneficial to heart health.

Day three: Flexibility and Balance Training.

On Day 3, the emphasis changes to flexibility and balance exercises to increase mobility, reduce joint stiffness, and boost proprioception.

• **Yoga or Tai Chi (30–45 minutes)** can enhance flexibility, balance, and stress reduction. Both techniques stimulate the mind and body, making them ideal for general health.

• **For standing leg lifts (3 sets of 12 reps per leg)**, stand on one leg and slowly lift the other to the side. This straightforward exercise improves balance and develops the muscles that surround your hips.

• **Hamstring Stretch (hold for 30 seconds, 3 sets)**: Regularly stretching your hamstrings can assist in preserving mobility, especially as they tighten with age.

For example, studies suggest that older persons who practice yoga or Tai Chi at least twice a week have a 55% lower chance of falling. These exercises promote muscle and mental coordination, which is essential for retaining independence.

Day four: Active recovery.

After three days of intense exertion, your body needs to rest and heal. This does not imply sitting around all day; **active recovery** is low-intensity movement that increases blood flow without overtaxing the muscles.

• **Gentle walking or swimming (20 to 30 minutes)** are low-impact activities that keep the body moving without hurting the muscles.

• **Foam rolling (10-15 minutes)**: Use a foam roller to massage sore or tight muscles, improving circulation and promoting muscle recovery.

Day 5: Strength training (upper body focus)

On Day 5, we resume strength training but focus on the **upper body**, specifically the muscles in the chest, shoulders, back, and arms.

- **Overhead Press (3 sets of 8-12 reps)**: This exercise targets the **shoulders** and **triceps**, and it can be performed with dumbbells or resistance bands.

- **Bent-Over Rows (3 sets of 8-10 reps)**: Work the **back muscles**, including the **latissimus dorsi** and **rhomboids**, as well as the **biceps**.

- **Use bicep curls (three sets of 12–15 reps)** to build arm strength.

- **Perform tricep dips (3 sets of 10-12 reps)** on a bench or sturdy chair to target the triceps.

Day 6: High-Intensity Interval Training (HIIT)

HIIT is one of the most effective methods for improving cardiovascular health and **burning fat** in a short amount of time. . HIIT involves alternating between periods of high-intensity effort and low-intensity recovery.

- **Sprint Intervals**: Begin with a **30-second sprint** followed by a **90-second stroll**. Repeat for **20 to 25 minutes.**

- **Bodyweight Circuit**: Perform **burpees, jump squats,** and **mountain climbers** for 30 seconds each, followed by 30 seconds of recovery. Repeat for 15–20 minutes.

Studies demonstrate that HIIT can boost **aerobic capacity** more than steady-state cardio, making it an excellent choice for both heart health and fat loss.

Day 7: Flexibility, Balance, and Restorative Movement.

As the week comes to a close, renew your focus on **mobility, flexibility,** and **balance**. This day provides a gentler exercise practice while still stimulating the muscles and joints.

- **Dynamic stretching (15-20 minutes):** Perform full-range-of-motion stretches to loosen tight areas, especially in the hips, shoulders, and hamstrings.

• **Balance Drills**: Stand on one leg or perform **heel-to-toe walking** to challenge your balance and proprioception.

.Tip: Use Day 7 to relax both physically and psychologically. **Deep breathing exercises** and **meditation** can help with recuperation and stress reduction.

This weekly program addresses all components of health—muscle strength, cardiovascular fitness, flexibility, and balance—that are critical for healthy aging. Each day focuses on different aspects to keep you strong, agile, and resilient. Adjust the exercises and intensity to your current fitness level, but remember that **consistency** is key. By following this plan on a regular basis, you will not only combat the physical symptoms of aging but also improve your quality of life long into your older years.

4-WEEK PROGRESSIVE WORKOUT PLAN: ACTION STEPS

The following four-week workout regimen is intended to gradually test your body, allowing you to develop strength, cardiovascular endurance, flexibility, and balance over time. It is designed to accommodate all fitness levels, from beginners to those with more experienced training routines. The plan's intensity will gradually rise over the course of the weeks, allowing your body to adapt and develop stronger without exceeding your system.

Week 1: Building a Foundation

Concentrate on developing a regimen, acquiring excellent form, and stimulating muscles without overexertion.

Day One: Strength Training (Full Body)

- **Squats (3 sets of 10 reps)**

- **Push-ups (3 sets of 8 reps)** (kneeling push-ups for beginners)

- **Deadlifts (3 sets of 8 reps)** (light dumbbells or bodyweight)

- **Plank (hold for 20 seconds, 3 sets)**

Day Two: Cardio

- **Brisk walking or light jogging (25 minutes)**
- **Cycling (20 minutes)**

Day three: Flexibility and Balance.

- **Yoga or Tai Chi (30 minutes)**
- **Hamstring stretches (3 sets of 30 seconds each leg)**
- **Standing leg lifts (2 sets of 10 reps per leg)**

Day four: Active recovery.

- **Gentle walking (20-25 minutes)**
- **Foam rolling (10 minutes)**

Day 5: Strength training (upper body)

- **Overhead press (3 sets of 8 reps with light weights)**
- **Bent-over rows (3 sets of 10 reps)**
- **Bicep curls (3 sets of 10 reps)**
- **Tricep dips (3 sets of 8 reps)**

Day Six: HIIT

- **Sprint intervals (20 seconds sprint, 40 seconds rest, 15 minutes)**
- **Bodyweight circuit (burpees, jump squats, mountain climbers for 20 seconds each, 2 rounds)**

Day 7: Flexibility, Balance, and Rest

- **Dynamic stretching (15 minutes)**
- **Balance drills (single-leg standing or heel-to-toe walking)**

Week 2: Increasing Intensity

In Week 2, begin to slightly increase the weight in strength exercises and the duration of your cardio sessions.

Day 1: Strength Training (Full Body)

- **Squats (3 sets of 12 reps)**
- **Push-ups (3 sets of 10 reps)**
- **Deadlifts (3 sets of 10 reps)**
- **Plank (hold for 30 seconds, 3 sets)**

Day 2: Cardio

- **Brisk walking or light jogging (30 minutes)**
- **Cycling (25 minutes)**

Day 3: Flexibility and Balance

- **Yoga (35 minutes)**
- **Hamstring stretches (3 sets of 45 seconds)**

- **Standing leg lifts (3 sets of 10 reps per leg)**

Day 4: Active Recovery

- **Gentle swimming (20-30 minutes)**
- **Foam rolling (15 minutes)**

Day 5: Strength Training (Upper Body)

- **Overhead press (3 sets of 10 reps)**
- **Bent-over rows (3 sets of 12 reps)**
- **Bicep curls (3 sets of 12 reps)**
- **Tricep dips (3 sets of 10 reps)**

Day 6: HIIT

- **Sprint intervals (25 seconds sprint, 45 seconds rest, 20 minutes)**
- **Bodyweight circuit (burpees, jump squats, mountain climbers for 30 seconds each, 3 rounds)**

Day 7: Flexibility, Balance, and Rest

- **Dynamic stretching (20 minutes)**
- **Balance drills (increase hold time on one leg)**

Week 3*:* Further Progression

By Week 3, the weights increase slightly for strength exercises, and HIIT sessions become longer.

Day 1: Strength Training (Full Body)

- **Squats (4 sets of 12 reps)**
- **Push-ups (4 sets of 12 reps)**
- **Deadlifts (4 sets of 12 reps)**
- **Plank (hold for 45 seconds, 4 sets)**

Day 2: Cardio

- **Brisk walking or jogging (35 minutes)**
- **Cycling (30 minutes)**

Day 3: Flexibility and Balance

- **Yoga (40 minutes)**
- **Hamstring stretches (4 sets of 45 seconds)**
- **Standing leg lifts (3 sets of 12 reps per leg)**

Day 4: Active Recovery

- **Gentle hiking or swimming (30 minutes)**
- **Foam rolling (15 minutes)**

Day 5: Strength Training (Upper Body)

- **Overhead press (4 sets of 12 reps)**
- **Bent-over rows (4 sets of 12 reps)**
- **Bicep curls (4 sets of 12 reps)**
- **Tricep dips (4 sets of 12 reps)**

Day 6: HIIT

- **Sprint intervals (30 seconds sprint, 30 seconds rest, 25 minutes)**

- **Bodyweight circuit (burpees, jump squats, mountain climbers for 40 seconds each, 4 rounds)**

Day 7: Flexibility, Balance, and Rest

- **Dynamic stretching (25 minutes)**
- **Balance drills (add small movements while balancing, like reaching forward)**

Week 4: Peak Challenge

In the final week, increase the intensity of strength and HIIT workouts, and aim to complete your sessions more efficiently.

Day 1: Strength Training (Full Body)

- **Squats (5 sets of 12 reps)**
- **Push-ups (5 sets of 12 reps)**
- **Deadlifts (5 sets of 12 reps)**

- **Plank (hold for 60 seconds, 4 sets)**

Day 2: Cardio

- **Brisk walking or jogging (40 minutes)**
- **Cycling (35 minutes)**

Day 3: Flexibility and Balance

- **Yoga (45 minutes)**
- **Hamstring stretches (4 sets of 60 seconds)**
- **Standing leg lifts (4 sets of 12 reps per leg)**

Day 4: Active Recovery

- **Gentle swimming or hiking (30-40 minutes)**
- **Foam rolling (15 minutes)**

Day 5: Strength Training (Upper Body)

- **Overhead press (5 sets of 12 reps)**
- **Bent-over rows (5 sets of 12 reps)**
- **Bicep curls (5 sets of 12 reps)**

- **Tricep dips (5 sets of 12 reps)**

Day 6: HIIT

- **Sprint intervals (30 seconds sprint, 30 seconds rest, 30 minutes)**
- **Bodyweight circuit (burpees, jump squats, mountain climbers for 45 seconds each, 4 rounds)**

Day 7: Flexibility, Balance, and Rest

- **Dynamic stretching (30 minutes)**
- **Balance drills (advanced movements like single-leg deadlifts for balance)**

Progressive adaptation at all levels

This **4-week progressive training routine** will gradually test your body. The progressive rise in intensity enables your muscles, heart, and joints to adjust safely, resulting in improved overall fitness and resilience. Whether you're a beginner hoping to get started with fitness or an established exerciser wishing to improve your routine, this plan can be tailored to your specific needs.

Chapter 7

Mental Health and Aging.

Cognitive decline and brain health: Understanding the aging brain.

Changes in our brains are as natural as graying hair or wrinkled skin as we become older. Cognitive aging impairs our ability to reason, learn, and remember. While many characteristics of mental sharpness, such as processing speed and working memory, normally deteriorate over time, it is crucial to recognize that these changes are not always indicative of disease. Instead, they are part of the natural aging process. Understanding the brain's intricate processes and participating in lifestyle modifications can help prevent cognitive decline and, in many situations, allow us to thrive mentally well into our senior years.

The Brain's Aging Process

To understand cognitive decline, we must first examine what occurs in the brain as we age. One of the most important parts of aging is the brain's neurons. Neurons are the brain's communication highways, delivering information across synapses that control everything from memory to motor skills. The number of neurons reduces with age, as does the overall volume of the brain. This process impacts cognitive skills such as memory retention, problem solving, and multitasking.

For example, research suggests that in our 30s and 40s, we begin to lose neurons in the hippocampus, which is crucial for memory formation and learning. By the time we are in our 70s or 80s, this steady loss may affect our ability to remember names, recent events, or where we left our keys.

Furthermore, blood supply to the brain decreases over time, limiting the oxygen and nutrients required for optimal brain function. Decreased blood flow can also cause damage to the brain's white matter, which are fiber tracts that connect distinct brain regions and hinder communication between them. This is frequently why older persons have slower processing times or take longer to learn new skills.

Why Cognitive Decline Isn't Inevitable: Brain Plasticity

While it may sound bleak, cognitive decline isn't inevitable. One of the most fascinating discoveries in neuroscience is the concept of neuroplasticity—the brain's astonishing ability to remodel itself, make new synaptic connections, and even generate new neurons via a process known as neurogenesis. Neuroplasticity implies that given the correct stimulus, our brains may adapt, grow, and maintain cognitive function throughout life.

For example, mentally stimulating activities such as learning a new language or playing musical instruments can boost neuroplasticity. According to research, frequent cognitive training, such as puzzles, memory games, or even difficult problem-solving tasks, might help strengthen brain resilience and prevent age-related deterioration.

A 2014 study published in The Lancet found that older persons who participated in cognitively stimulating activities had a 29% lower risk of dementia than those who led less mentally active lifestyles.

Mental health and cognitive decline: How stress accelerates aging.

Our mental health has a significant impact on the aging brain, in addition to biological processes. Chronic stress, despair, and anxiety can all hasten cognitive loss by causing inflammation in the brain and raising cortisol levels, the body's principal stress hormone. Prolonged exposure to elevated cortisol levels is harmful to the hippocampus, causing memory impairments and increasing the risk of dementia. A study conducted by the University of California discovered that people with high cortisol levels had faster losses in brain capacity and cognitive function over time. Those who had long-term depression were more likely to have evidence of cognitive impairment early in life.

Practical Strategies for Protecting Your Brain as You Age.

1. **Diet and Nutrition**: One of the most effective ways to promote brain health is through eating. Foods high in antioxidants, omega-3 fatty acids, and other anti-inflammatory chemicals protect brain cells from harm.

The Mediterranean diet, which includes fruits, vegetables, whole grains, and healthy fats such as olive oil, has been associated with improved cognitive performance and a lower risk of Alzheimer's disease. A study published in the journal Neurology found that older persons who followed the Mediterranean diet had slower rates of cognitive deterioration than those who followed normal Western diets.

2. **Exercise**: Physical activity is one of the most effective strategies to maintain brain health. Exercise boosts

blood flow to the brain, stimulates neurogenesis, and helps avoid the accumulation of toxic proteins that can lead to neurodegenerative illnesses. A 2018 study published by the American Academy of Neurology discovered that regular aerobic exercise can increase the size of the hippocampus, hence improving memory and slowing cognitive decline. Even basic exercises such as walking or swimming for 30 minutes every day can provide long-term brain benefits.

3. **Sleep Hygiene**: Sleep is crucial for cognitive function. Toxins that accumulate during the day are removed from the brain during sleep. Chronic sleep deprivation has been associated with memory loss, emotional issues, and an increased risk of Alzheimer's disease. Studies have found that persons who routinely obtain less than six hours of sleep every night are more likely to experience brain aging, decreased cognitive performance, and accelerated memory loss.

4. **Social Engagement**: Staying socially active can help reduce emotions of loneliness and sadness, both of which are associated with cognitive decline. Strong social interactions stimulate the brain and keep cognitive abilities sharp. In a landmark study, older persons who frequently participated in social activities and maintained friendships had a 70% lower risk of dementia than those who were more socially isolated.

COGNITIVE LONGEVITY: IT'S NEVER TOO LATE TO START

The message is that, although aging is unavoidable, cognitive decline is not. Adopting a brain-healthy lifestyle can dramatically reduce the effects of aging on the brain. Whether you're in your 30s or your 70s, it's never too late to prioritize your mental health. Investing in your mental health now will ensure a brighter, more robust brain in the future.

Living vibrantly as we age is about more than just our physical health; it's about keeping our minds sharp, staying engaged, and embracing lifelong learning. Cognitive longevity is within grasp, and research suggests that taking even little steps toward mental well-being can add years of clarity and joy to our lives.

Mindfulness and meditation can reduce stress and promote neuroplasticity.

Aging is a complex process that affects both the body and the psyche. As we become older, stress management becomes increasingly important in preserving brain health and preventing age-related cognitive decline. Mindfulness and meditation, two ancient techniques, have proven to be effective strategies for stress reduction, mental well-being, and neuroplasticity. In this section, we'll look at how these routines help maintain and even improve cognitive performance as we age.

The Science of Stress and Cognitive Decline

Chronic stress is one of the most damaging elements to brain function, particularly as we age. It causes the release of cortisol, a hormone that, in modest amounts, aids the body's response to urgent dangers. However, prolonged exposure to increased cortisol levels, which are common in persons suffering from chronic stress, can harm crucial brain regions such as the hippocampus and prefrontal cortex. These sections are in charge of memory, mood control, and decision-making. As a result, prolonged stress hastens brain aging, contributing to memory loss, anxiety, and an increased risk of neurodegenerative disorders such as Alzheimer's.

For example, Harvard Medical School research showed that patients who endure continuous stress have higher levels of cognitive impairment and are more likely to develop dementia. High cortisol levels have been demonstrated to atrophy the hippocampus, impairing learning and memory.

Mindfulness and Meditation: What Are They?

Mindfulness is the practice of being completely present in the moment, paying attention to your thoughts, feelings, and bodily sensations without passing judgment. This awareness directs attention to the present moment rather than concentrating on the past or worrying about the future.

Meditation, on the other hand, is a broader set of practices that includes mindfulness as well as focused attention on a specific object, idea, or activity (for example, breathing). Both mindfulness and meditation seek to calm the mind, alleviate stress, and build a stronger connection with oneself.

How mindfulness and meditation reduce stress

Mindfulness and meditation directly reduce the detrimental effects of stress by activating the parasympathetic nerve system, sometimes known as the "rest and digest" system. When the parasympathetic system is triggered, cortisol levels fall, heart rate drops, and the body relaxes. This physiological shift promotes healing and decreases the damage that prolonged stress brings to the brain and body.

A study published in Psychiatry Research indicated that participants in an 8-week mindfulness-based stress reduction (MBSR) program had significant reductions in both psychological stress and cortisol levels. This decrease in stress indicators coincided with a rise in gray matter density in the hippocampus, the brain region responsible for learning and memory.

Promoting Neuroplasticity: Developing a Resilient Brain

One of the most striking advantages of mindfulness and meditation is their potential to enhance **neuroplasticity**—the brain's ability to reshape itself by generating new neural connections over time. Neuroplasticity is critical for cognitive longevity because it allows us to keep learning, adapt to new difficulties, and recover from cognitive setbacks, such as brain injury or age-related decline.

Meditation promotes neuroplasticity by thickening the cerebral cortex, especially in areas associated with attention and sensory processing. This keeps the brain nimble, helping it to integrate new information and recover more quickly from disturbances. Furthermore, mindfulness lessens the consequences of mental "clutter" that can overload the brain and impair cognitive ability as we age.

In a groundbreaking study from the University of California, researchers discovered that people who practiced mindfulness meditation for just 12 minutes per day for 8 weeks had increased activity in the default mode network (DMN), which is involved in daydreaming, self-reflection, and memory processing. Increased DMN activity is linked to improved cognitive performance and memory retention, especially in elderly persons.

Mindfulness and Memory: Slowing Cognitive Decline

Mindfulness and meditation are especially beneficial at improving **working memory**—the brain's ability to store and handle information in real time. According to research, meditation can delay or even reverse this cognitive decline, which begins with aging.

A research study from the University of Wisconsin-Madison found that older persons who practiced mindfulness meditation for just 15 minutes per day for 8 weeks had a significant increase in working memory. This benefit lasted even six months after the trial finished, implying that mindfulness can "train" the brain to better manage information over time.

Practical applications: bringing mindfulness and meditation into everyday life

1. **Daily Meditation Practice**: Even short sessions of meditation (10 to 15 minutes per day) can have a significant impact on stress reduction and cognitive wellness. Start with simple mindfulness exercises, such as focusing on your breathing or scanning your body for stress. Use guided meditation applications like Calm or Headspace to help organize your practice. These

applications include a number of meditation options, including mindfulness, loving-kindness, and body-scan meditations, to meet a variety of needs.

2. **Mindful eating** is one method to bring mindfulness into your daily life. Slowing down and focusing on the flavors, textures, and sensations of your meal might help you avoid overeating, improve digestion, and build a healthier relationship with food—all while supporting brain health.

3. **Mental Movement**: Yoga and Tai Chi combine physical movement and mental awareness, making them excellent activities for brain and body wellness. These activities improve balance, flexibility, and coordination while lowering stress and increasing neuroplasticity.

For example, research published in the Journal of Alzheimer's Disease indicated that seniors who engaged in mindful movement techniques such as Tai Chi had lower rates of cognitive deterioration than those who did not.

4. **Mindful Listening**: During conversations, be fully present and attentive to the speaker without interrupting or planning your response. This style of listening strengthens social relationships, lowers stress, and improves brain function.

Incorporating mindfulness and meditation into our everyday routines is one of the most effective ways to maintain mental health and increase cognitive resilience. By lowering stress and encouraging neuroplasticity, these techniques reduce the aging process and protect against age-related cognitive loss. Science is gradually verifying what ancient wisdom has long known: our brains are pliable, and how we interact with the world has a substantial impact on our mental health.

Whether you're just getting started or want to improve your practice, meditation and mindfulness provide long-term mental health advantages. It is never too late to train your brain and improve its ability to thrive, regardless of age.

EMOTIONAL RESILIENCE: MANAGING THE CHALLENGES OF AGING

Aging, like other life stages, has its own distinct emotional landscape. As we get older, we confront a variety of emotional issues, including retirement, loss of loved ones, and changes in our self-image. Despite their negative effects on our mental health, these issues do not have to lower our quality of life. In fact, developing and maintaining emotional resilience is critical to not only surviving but also thriving in the face of these challenges.

Emotional resilience is the capacity to adapt, cope, and recover from stress, adversity, and trauma. It is not about avoiding terrible situations but about developing the mental and emotional tools to deal with them. In this chapter, we will look at how emotional resilience can help us confront aging with grace and courage, as well as techniques to aid.

Understanding the Emotional Challenges of Aging

• Retirement and loss of purpose

Retirement can be a double-edged sword. On the one hand, it can be liberating—time to travel, pursue hobbies, and unwind after years of hard work. On the other hand, it might result in feelings of purposelessness or even depression. Many people get their sense of identity and self-worth from their jobs. When that function disappears, they may struggle to find new purpose in their life.

For example, a 2016 study published in the Journal of Aging & Health discovered that those who retired without a clear sense of purpose were more likely to experience emotional distress and depressive symptoms than those who developed new objectives or interests. Those who took on new tasks, such as volunteering or learning new skills, reported greater life satisfaction after retirement.

Emotional resilience at this stage entails reinventing meaning, whether through hobbies, social involvement, or new duties. Your work becomes less important than your fulfillment.

• Dealing with loss and grief

Aging often brings the awful reality of losing loved ones, whether they are spouses, friends, or family members. Grief is a severe emotional struggle that can lead to emotions of loneliness, misery, and despair. While the agony of loss never fully goes away, emotional resilience is the ability to manage that pain while still living a meaningful life.

In her book On Grief and Grieving, Elisabeth Kübler-Ross uses the stages of grief—denial, anger, bargaining, depression, and acceptance—to help readers comprehend the emotional process of loss. These stages are not sequential, but they do provide a framework for working through sorrow. Emotional resilience enables people to acknowledge their sadness, embrace their emotions, and discover new ways to participate with life.

Learning appropriate grief processing techniques is essential for developing emotional resilience in the face of loss. Whether through counseling, support groups, or relying on personal relationships, it is critical to make room for emotional recovery. The idea is to go forward rather than "move on".

• Changes in self-image and physical appearance

Our physical appearance and abilities evolve organically as we age. For many people, this might result in a crisis of self-image or self-esteem, especially in a society that celebrates youth and energy. Aging can cause wrinkles, gray hair, weight changes, and decreased mobility, making people feel less confident or even invisible.

A 2017 study in the International Journal of Behavioral Medicine discovered that older persons who internalized negative aging stereotypes (such as equating old age with weakness or ineptitude) had higher levels of anxiety, sadness, and cognitive deterioration. Those who saw aging as an opportunity for wisdom and progress, on the other hand, reported improved mental health and cognitive function.

Reframing our perception of aging helps us develop emotional resilience. Focusing on the positives, like knowledge and experience, can change our self-image from loss to progress and gratitude. Regular self-compassion techniques, such as mindfulness and self-affirmation, can also boost self-esteem.

Strategies for Developing Emotional Resilience in Aging

1. **Develop social bonds**

One of the most effective ways to develop emotional resilience is to maintain strong social connections. Research has consistently demonstrated that those who keep close friendships and family ties fare better with the emotional problems of aging. These ties offer a support system to rely on during times of stress, loss, or transition.

The Harvard Study of Adult Development, which followed people for more than 80 years, found that the quality of social ties was the single most important predictor of emotional and physical well-being in later life. Those who maintained strong social relationships lived longer, had fewer cases of dementia, and reported higher levels of enjoyment.

Regular interaction with family, friends, or community groups promotes emotional resiliency. Staying socially engaged, whether through volunteer work, club membership, or simply retaining close friendships, provides emotional support and a sense of belonging.

2. **Develop a growth mindset**

Psychologist Carol Dweck's concept of the "growth mindset" suggests that persons who believe their talents may improve through effort and learning are more likely to overcome problems. This perspective is especially important in later life, since it can help people stay open to new experiences, learn from their mistakes, and see setbacks (like retirement or physical deterioration) as opportunities for growth rather than fixed impediments.

In a 2020 study published in Psychological Science, researchers discovered that older persons with a growth mindset are better able to recuperate from stress and adapt to changing situations, such as physical restrictions or life transitions. They exhibited stronger psychological resilience than those with a fixed attitude, who saw aging as a downhill spiral.

Adopting a growth mindset promotes resilience. Rather than seeing age as a period of unavoidable decline, emotionally resilient people see it as an opportunity for continual learning, flexibility, and self-development.

3. Practice mindfulness and acceptance

Mindfulness, or paying attention to the present moment without judgment, has been shown to dramatically improve emotional resilience. By focusing on the now, people can lessen their anxiety about the future and accept the changes that come with age. Acceptance does not imply giving up but rather acknowledging reality as it is and deciding how best to proceed.

Researchers at the University of California, Los Angeles (UCLA) discovered that older persons who practiced mindfulness had reduced levels of stress and anxiety and were better able to cope with life changes. They also demonstrated greater emotional stability and positivity.

Regular mindfulness meditation, as well as simple practices such as deep breathing and grounding exercises, can help reduce stress and increase emotional resilience. These strategies promote acceptance and offer tools for coping with the ups and downs of aging.

Emotional resilience is a lifelong skill

Building emotional resilience is a continual process that gets increasingly important as we age. Whether dealing with retirement, grief, changes in self-image, or other problems, emotional resilience enables us to adapt and thrive. The key to emotional resilience is how we perceive and respond to life's inevitable challenges—by cultivating social relationships, having a development mindset, and practicing mindfulness, we may age gracefully and with strength.

ACTION STEP: DAILY MINDFULNESS PRACTICES AND JOURNALING PROMPTS FOR MENTAL CLARITY AND EMOTIONAL WELLBEING

Integrating mindfulness and journaling into your daily practice can greatly improve mental clarity and emotional resilience, particularly as we age. A planned action plan is provided below, along with easy mindfulness techniques and journaling prompts to assist you in focusing your thoughts, processing emotions, and cultivating a sense of peace and balance.

Daily Mindfulness Practices

1. Morning Breathing Meditation (5-10 minutes).

Start the day with a quick, focused breathing practice. Sit in a comfortable position, close your eyes, and take deep breaths in through your nose and out slowly through your mouth. Focus on your breathing rhythm and body sensations on each inhale and exhale.

- **Objective**: To start the day with mental clarity, setting a calm and focused tone for the rest of the day.

• When ideas come, softly return your focus to your breathing without judgment.

Tip: For guided breathing exercises, try apps like Calm or Headspace.

2. **Midday Mindful Walking (10-15 Minutes)**

Take a little walk in the middle of the day. Concentrate on the sensation of your feet touching the ground, the sounds surrounding you, and the things you see. Be completely present in the process of walking, not allowing your attention to wander to distractions or problems.

• **Objective**: Break up the day with mindful exercise to reduce stress and increase awareness.

• if your mind wanders to duties or anxieties, slowly refocus on walking sensations.

3. Evening Body Scan Meditation (10–15 minutes)

To relieve stress, practice a body scan meditation before going to bed. Lie down or sit comfortably and mentally scan your entire body, head to toe. Identify any places of tightness or discomfort and visualize releasing them with each inhalation.

• **Objective**: To prepare your body and mind for restful sleep by promoting relaxation.

• **Example**: Imagine each area of tension softening as you breathe, allowing your body to fully relax into the present moment.

Journal prompts for emotional well-being

1. Daily Gratitude.

Every morning or evening, jot down three things you are grateful for. This could be as simple as a decent cup of coffee or as important as spending time with loved ones.

- **Objective:** Increase emotional resilience by cultivating a positive mentality and focusing on the positive aspects of life.

- **Prompt**: "Today, I am thankful for..."

2. Processing Emotions

When you're feeling overwhelmed, apprehensive, or stressed, record your thoughts and feelings in a stream-of-consciousness format. Allow your emotions to spill onto the page, without regard for syntax or organization.

- **Objective:** To clear mental clutter and acquire insight into your emotional condition, facilitating the processing of challenging emotions.

- **Prompt:** "I am currently feeling... because..."

3. Reflecting on Challenges and Growth

Consider how you handled problems at the end of the week. Consider how you might continue to develop emotional resilience and learn from these experiences.

- **Objective:** Foster a growth attitude by viewing problems as opportunities for personal progress.

- **Ask yourself:** "This week, I faced the following challenge... and I learned that..."

4. Mindful Moment Journal

Write about a time in your day when you felt fully present. Describe your actions, emotions, and observations.

- **Objective:** Improve mindfulness awareness and integration into daily routines.

- **Prompt:** "Today, I felt completely present when..."

Building Emotional Resilience with Mindfulness and Journaling

These daily mindfulness techniques and journaling prompts aim to improve emotional well-being and mental clarity by encouraging you to be present and reflect on your experiences. Regular mindfulness and journaling practice will help you relax, reduce stress, and develop your emotional resilience. This action step provides a solid foundation for managing the emotional problems of aging, helping you to face life's transformations with grace and confidence.

Chapter 8

Lifestyle Habits That Promote Longevity

Aging is unavoidable, yet how we age is primarily determined by our everyday behaviors. The decisions we make—from what we eat to how we move—can either accelerate or halt the aging process, keeping us healthier for longer. **Sleep** is an often-overlooked but vital component of this equation. Sleep is more than just a rest period; it is also a time of crucial repair and restoration, during which our bodies engage in a variety of processes that protect our physical and mental health.

However, not all sleep is equal. Many of us are unknowingly reducing the quality of our sleep, denying our bodies the opportunity to recover and recharge. In this chapter, we'll look at why sleep is crucial for longevity, how it affects cellular repair, brain function, and emotional well-being, and, most significantly, how we can improve our sleep habits to slow the passage of time.

1. SLEEP AND AGING: THE FOUNTAIN OF YOUTH IS HIDDEN IN PLAIN SIGHT

As we get older, our bodies lose part of their natural ability to recuperate from regular stresses. This is where sleep comes in as a powerful ally. Every night, during deep sleep, our bodies enter a state of regeneration, rebuilding damaged tissues and regaining cognitive function. It's no coincidence that poor sleep has been connected to a variety of age-related ailments, including heart disease, dementia, and diabetes. Sleep is essential for cellular repair because it allows our cells to recuperate from oxidative stress, reduces inflammation, and stimulates the production of growth hormones that promote muscle and bone health.

Lack of adequate sleep is essentially hastening the aging process. Sleep deprivation has been proven in studies to shorten telomeres, which are the protective caps at the ends of our DNA strands and critical markers of aging. When telomeres shorten, cells become more susceptible to malfunction, raising the risk of chronic illness and premature aging. In other words, the longer and better you sleep, the higher your chances of aging gracefully.

However, achieving deep, restorative sleep requires more than just eight hours per night. This is where **sleep hygiene** comes in—a series of habits that promote healthy sleep patterns. Let's look at the precise behaviors that can improve your sleep for life.

Sleep Hygiene: Simple Tips to Improve Your Sleep Quality

Just as we care for our physical and mental health through nutrition and exercise, effective sleep hygiene is critical for attaining the quality sleep required for long-term health. While individual sleep needs differ, the basics of sleep hygiene are universal. Simple changes, such as establishing a relaxing environment or controlling your nighttime routines, can have a significant impact on your sleep quality.

• **Establish a Consistent Sleep Schedule:** The body's circadian rhythm regulates sleep and wake cycles. Going to bed and waking up at the same time every day helps synchronize the clock, resulting in more peaceful sleep.

• **Make your bedroom a sleep-inducing environment**. Keep everything cool, dark, and quiet. Light exposure, particularly blue light from screens, interferes with the generation of melatonin, a hormone that regulates sleep. Using blackout curtains, white noise generators, or eye masks can improve your sleeping conditions.

• **Limit stimulants before bedtime,** as caffeine, nicotine, and alcohol can disrupt sleep cycles. While alcohol may temporarily make you drowsy, it interferes with the deep sleep stages required for physical and mental healing. Try not to consume these things four to six hours before bedtime.

• **Set a relaxing pre-sleep routine** to inform your body that it's time for sleep. Reading, meditating, or having a warm bath are all excellent relaxation activities.

• **Limit heavy meals before bedtime** to avoid disrupting sleep due to digestion and discomfort.

2. INTERMITTENT FASTING AND CALORIE RESTRICTION HAVE SCIENTIFIC BENEFITS FOR ANTI-AGING AND LONGEVITY.

Fasting, in its different forms, has been done for ages, frequently as a spiritual or religious ritual. However, science now suggests that intermittent fasting (IF) and calorie restriction (CR) may hold the secret to reducing the aging process and increasing longevity. Both treatments focus on reducing calorie intake, but they differ in how they are implemented—intermittent fasting requires particular eating and fasting windows, whereas caloric restriction focuses on reducing overall daily caloric intake while maintaining nutrition.

The Science of Fasting and Longevity

A number of factors contribute to cellular aging, including oxidative stress, inflammation, and DNA damage. Fasting appears to inhibit several of these processes by activating a variety of defensive mechanisms. Intermittent fasting and caloric restriction have been demonstrated in studies to enhance animal lifetime, and new research suggests that people may benefit as well.

Autophagy Activation

Fasting induces autophagy, a type of cellular housekeeping system. When the body goes into a fasting state, cells begin to break down damaged or defective components, recycling them to produce energy. This process is necessary for maintaining healthy cells and tissues and may reduce age-related cellular decline. In animal models, greater autophagy has been associated with longer lifespans and protection against neurodegenerative illnesses such as Alzheimer's.

Insulin Sensitivity and Metabolic Health

Both intermittent fasting and caloric restriction enhance insulin sensitivity, which is especially important as we age. As our bodies grow less efficient at processing glucose, we are more likely to acquire type 2 diabetes. Fasting helps manage blood sugar and improve insulin responses, which promote metabolic health and may protect against age-related illnesses like diabetes, obesity, and cardiovascular disease. Fasting also lowers IGF-1 (Insulin-like Growth Factor), a hormone that, in excess, promotes aging and cancer.

Reducing inflammation and oxidative stress

Fasting has been shown to lower inflammation, which is a major contributor to chronic disease and aging. It reduces oxidative stress by lowering the levels of reactive oxygen species (ROS), which are chemicals that cause DNA and cellular damage. Reduced inflammation and oxidative stress not only protect your organs but also boost brain health, potentially lowering your risk of cognitive decline and Alzheimer's disease.

Intermittent Fasting Approaches

There are various popular methods for practicing intermittent fasting, each with its own structure:

1. **The 16/8 method** entails fasting for 16 hours and eating all meals within an 8-hour timeframe. For example, you might eat between midday and 8 p.m., missing breakfast but eating regularly during that time.

2. **The 5:2 Diet**: On this regimen, you eat normally five days a week and dramatically limit your calorie consumption to around 500-600 calories the remaining two days.

3. **Alternate-Day Fasting**: This method involves alternating between days of normal eating and days when you eat very little or nothing at all.

Each of these strategies is adaptable, making it easier for people to choose a fasting regimen that suits their lifestyle and particular health goals. According to research, intermittent fasting may replicate some of the benefits of caloric restriction without the requirement for constant calorie reduction, making it a more sustainable alternative for many people.

3. CALORIE RESTRICTION: A LONG-TERM APPROACH

Calorie restriction (CR), on the other hand, is limiting total calorie consumption by 20-30% while still absorbing necessary nutrients. The goal of CR is to slow down metabolic activities and minimize the damage produced by oxidative stress and free radicals. Long-term calorie restriction has been found to enhance lifespan in a variety of animals, ranging from yeast to rodents, and is associated with a lower risk of numerous age-related disorders, such as cancer, cardiovascular disease, and diabetes.

The Caloric Restriction Society's Biosphere 2 Experiment, a landmark study, proved CR's dramatic effects on human health indices. Participants who followed a low-calorie diet exhibited benefits in cholesterol, blood pressure, insulin sensitivity, and inflammatory markers—all of which are important for aging well.

However, it is crucial to remember that caloric restriction must be done cautiously, with an adequate intake of vitamins, minerals, and proteins to prevent malnutrition. Proper meal planning and a balanced diet play a crucial part in maximizing the effects of CR while maintaining overall health.

Real-world examples and implementations

Consider the **Blue Zones**—regions where people live longer than the average, such as Okinawa, Japan, and Sardinia, Italy. Many people in these places practice calorie restriction and fasting on a natural basis, whether through dietary or cultural activities. In Okinawa, for example, the notion of **Hara Hachi Bu**, or eating until 80% full, is a sort of natural caloric restriction.

In modern times, people have embraced intermittent fasting patterns that offer considerable health benefits. For example, Dr. Valter Longo's **Fasting Mimicking Diet** (FMD) has shown promise in promoting longevity by replicating the benefits of fasting while allowing for calorie restriction, making it easier to follow.

The Longevity Advantages of Fasting and Caloric Restriction

Intermittent fasting and caloric restriction are more than simply ways to lose weight; they are effective tactics for slowing aging, improving metabolic health, and increasing longevity. Reducing calorie intake, whether through fasting periods or total dietary adjustments, allows your body to participate in processes such as autophagy, increase insulin sensitivity, and reduce inflammation—all of which are essential for graceful aging.

Incorporating these habits into your lifestyle, even in tiny ways, may open the possibility of not just living a longer but also a better, more vibrant life. The evidence is clear: a thoughtful approach to eating, whether through fasting or calorie restriction, is the key to unlocking the body's innate longevity mechanisms.

4. SOCIAL CONNECTIONS: THE EFFECT OF RELATIONSHIPS ON HEALTH AND AGING

Strong social relationships are beneficial not just to our emotional well-being but also to our physical health and lifespan. Numerous studies have found that having close, supportive relationships can dramatically extend life, lower the risk of chronic diseases, and improve mental health as we age. In fact, social isolation has been related to a variety of unfavorable health consequences, making it just as important a risk factor for premature mortality as smoking or obesity.

The Science of Social Connection and Longevity

As we get older, the quality and amount of our social connections become more crucial in shaping our later lives. According to research, persons with strong social networks—whether through family, friends, or community involvement—live longer and have better overall health.

Reduced stress and inflammation

Positive social ties help reduce stress's negative consequences. Chronic stress can hasten aging by inducing inflammation and cellular damage. Social contacts, particularly those that promote emotional support, aid in the reduction of stress hormones such as cortisol, which, over time, can lead to lower inflammation and enhanced immunological function.

A **2009 study** published in the journal Health Psychology discovered that those with larger social networks and more regular social interactions had lower levels of systemic inflammation, which is a major cause of many age-related disorders such as heart disease, diabetes, and dementia.

Cardiovascular Health

Social support also has a significant impact on cardiovascular health. According to studies, persons who maintain close connections are less likely to develop cardiovascular disease. Loneliness and social isolation, on the other hand, have been linked to elevated blood pressure, greater levels of circulating stress hormones, and an increased risk of developing coronary artery disease.

The **Harvard Study** of Adult Development, which studied participants for almost 80 years, found that persons with stronger social bonds lived longer and healthier lives. One of the study's main results was that intimate relationships, rather than money or celebrity, are what keep individuals content and healthy throughout their lives, and that solid relationships safeguard both mental and physical health.

Mental health and cognitive function

Social involvement is also important for cognitive wellness. As we age, our cognitive function may diminish, but maintaining social relationships can serve as a buffer against these changes. Social contacts increase mental activity, which keeps the brain engaged and promotes neuroplasticity (the brain's ability to establish and reorganize connections).

For example, those who have a lot of social support are less likely to develop dementia or Alzheimer's disease. Conversations, games, or simply being among others can increase brain activity, resulting in improved cognitive function and a delay in the onset of age-related deterioration.

Longevity in Blue Zones

One common thread across the world's **Blue Zones**, or towns with the highest numbers of centenarians, is the presence of close-knit, supportive social networks. These locations, which include Okinawa, Japan, and Ikaria, Greece, value community living, intergenerational support, and everyday social engagement, all of which contribute to their unusual lifespan. In Okinawa, for example, people form lifelong social organizations known as "moais," which offer emotional and financial support throughout their lives. This sense of belonging and purpose promotes longer and healthier lives.

Combating loneliness among aging populations

While the value of social interactions is evident, the risk of isolation grows as people age. Retirement, the death of a spouse, or children moving away can all contribute to loneliness among older folks. However, developing and maintaining relationships—whether by volunteering, joining neighborhood groups, or staying in touch with family—can dramatically improve quality of life.

Senior centers, group activities, and virtual social platforms have been demonstrated to boost emotional well-being, reduce depression, and even increase life expectancy.

Relationships Can Help You Live Longer

Social ties are one of the most effective predictors of health as we age. Staying connected with people has been shown to reduce stress and inflammation while also enhancing heart and brain health. Nurturing relationships, whether through tight family attachments, friendships, or engagement in community activities, is equally crucial to longevity as food and exercise.

Action Step: Habit Tracker for Longevity

To achieve significant lifestyle changes, it is critical to develop habits that are both practical and sustainable. Here's a **habit tracker** that promotes consistency in three areas: **better sleep, intermittent fasting/eating windows**, and **nurturing relationships**. To measure success on a daily basis, you can either write a basic table in your journal or use digital software such as Google Sheets or a habit-tracking app.

1. Sleep Improvement Tracker

Goal: Get 7-9 hours of restful sleep per night to promote cellular regeneration and mental clarity.

Day's bedtime (target: 10 PM)

Sleep Duration (Target: Sleep for 7–9 hours)

Hygiene Practice (Yes or No)

Monday

Tuesday

Wednesday

Thursday

Friday

Saturday

Sunday

Sleep Hygiene Practices

• Reduce screen time 1 hour before bed.

• Limit caffeine after midday.

•Establish a calming bedtime routine, including meditation and reading.

• Optimize sleep quality by keeping the bedroom cold and dark.

2. Intermittent Fasting/Eating Windows Tracker

Goal: Use an intermittent fasting program (e.g., 16/8 or 5:2) to improve metabolic health and longevity.

Fasting Window Start Time

Fasting Window End time

Achieved 16/8 or 5:2? (Yes/No)

Monday

Tuesday

Wednesday

Thursday

Friday

Saturday

Sunday

Fasting tips:

• Only consume water, tea, or black coffee during fasting periods.

• Prioritize nutrient-dense meals during eating windows.

• Prioritize plant-based and healthy foods over processed options.

3. Relationship and Social Connections Tracker

Goal: Engage in meaningful social contacts every day to improve emotional and physical health.

Social Interaction (Type and Duration)

Nurtured relationship? (Yes/No)

Impact on mood/health (1–10)

Monday

Tuesday

Wednesday

Thursday

Friday

Saturday

Sunday

Ideas for Social Connections:

• Contact or meet with a friend or family member.

• Participate in group activities, clubs, or classes.

• Volunteer in your community.

• Engage in everyday, brief discussions to sustain social engagement.

Regularly recording these behaviors will allow you to understand how constant effort leads to benefits in health, mood, and longevity. Customize the tracker to fit your calendar, and remember to reflect on areas that need to be adjusted or prioritized on a weekly basis!

Chapter 9

Common Supplements for Graceful Aging.

As we go into the world of anti-aging supplements, it's vital to remember that, while they can help you live longer and age more slowly, they are not miracle cures. The trick is to use them in conjunction with a healthy lifestyle. Below, we'll look at some of the most researched and promising supplements for graceful aging, as supported by scientific evidence.

1. Vitamin D, the Sunshine Vitamin for Longevity.

• Vitamin D promotes bone density, muscle function, and immunological health. As we age, our ability to produce vitamin D from sunshine declines, increasing the risk of deficiency. Low vitamin D levels have been related to osteoporosis, heart disease, and even cognitive loss.

• Vitamin D promotes calcium absorption, which is crucial for maintaining bone density and reducing fractures in older persons.

Vitamin D deficiency has been related to increased susceptibility to infections, such as respiratory disorders. This is especially crucial for older persons, as the immune system weakens with age.

A 2019 study published in The American Journal of Clinical Nutrition found that senior people with adequate vitamin D levels had a considerably lower risk of falls and fractures, which are critical for maintaining independence and mobility in old life.

The recommended daily dosage is 1,000 to 2,000 IU, depending on blood levels, age, and sunshine exposure.

2. Resveratrol: The Anti-Aging Powerhouse

Resveratrol is a polyphenol present in red wine, grapes, and some berries. It's well-known for its ability to activate **Sirtuin 1**, a gene connected to lifespan and the regulation of cellular processes associated with aging. Resveratrol may reduce cellular aging by replicating the effects of calorie restriction, a well-known anti-aging therapy.

• Resveratrol promotes cell health by protecting against oxidative stress, which can cause DNA damage and aging. It may help improve mitochondrial activity, keeping your cells energized and efficient.

• This polyphenol can promote cardiovascular health by lowering inflammation and preventing arterial damage.

For example, animal studies have suggested that resveratrol can extend life by increasing mitochondrial function and lowering inflammation; however, human research is still ongoing.

The recommended daily dosage is 150-500 mg, while greater amounts may be used under medical supervision. For personalized advice, see a healthcare expert.

3. NAD+ Boosters: Supporting Cellular Energy

NAD+ (Nicotinamide Adenine Dinucleotide) is a coenzyme found in all cells in the body that aids in energy production and DNA repair. As we age, our NAD+ levels gradually fall, which is linked to the aging process and many age-related disorders.

• NAD+ promotes cellular repair and longevity by activating sirtuin enzymes that repair DNA and regulate genes. Low NAD+ levels have been linked to mitochondrial malfunction and metabolic diseases that occur with age.

• NAD+ protects neurons against oxidative stress, which can lead to neurodegenerative illnesses like Alzheimer's and Parkinson's.

Animal studies show that increasing NAD+ levels may help postpone the onset of age-related disorders, improve cognitive performance, and promote a longer life. Human clinical trials have demonstrated benefits in metabolic health and muscle function.

Recommended Supplements: **Nicotinamide Riboside (NR)** and **Nicotinamide Mononucleotide (NMN)** are common NAD+ boosters. Dosage recommendations vary, but normal doses range from 250 to 500 mg per day.

4. Omega-3 Fatty Acids: Anti-inflammatory Power

Omega-3 fatty acids, including EPA (eicosapentaenoic acid) and DHA (docosahexaenoic acid), are necessary lipids that have potent anti-inflammatory characteristics. Chronic inflammation contributes significantly to age-related disorders such as heart disease, arthritis, and Alzheimer's.

• Omega-3s promote **heart health** by lowering triglycerides, lowering blood pressure, and improving heart rhythm. These benefits are more important as we age.

• DHA is crucial for **brain function** and may lessen the risk of cognitive decline and Alzheimer's disease.

For example, a major meta-analysis published in JAMA discovered that regular omega-3 supplementation lowered the incidence of heart attacks, strokes, and mortality from heart disease in older persons.

Indicated dosage: 1,000-2,000 mg of EPA and DHA mixed daily, with greater doses indicated for patients with heart disease or inflammatory disorders.

5. Coenzyme Q10: Energize Your Cells

Coenzyme Q10 (CoQ10) is an antioxidant that helps cells produce energy, notably in the mitochondria. CoQ10 levels fall with age, which can lead to decreased energy, muscle weakness, and an increased risk of heart disease.

• CoQ10 is advised for older persons with cardiac issues, such as **heart failure** or **high blood pressure**, as it improves the heart's pumping efficiency.

• CoQ10 supplements can boost **energy**, reduce fatigue, and maintain muscle function in older persons.

A study published in The Journal of Aging Research discovered that CoQ10 supplementation in combination with selenium dramatically reduced mortality in older people with heart disease over a 10-year period.

Recommended Dosage: 100-300 mg per day, with a fat-containing meal for maximum absorption.

Creating a Personalized Supplement Routine

Supplements can be an effective adjunct to an anti-aging program, but they should not replace a healthy lifestyle. Incorporating proven supplements such as Vitamin D, resveratrol, NAD+ boosters, omega-3s, and CoQ10 into your daily routine can provide your body with the resources it requires to perform optimally as you age. ***Individual needs can vary depending on genetics, lifestyle, and health status, so always speak with a*** *healthcare practitioner before implementing a supplement plan*.

FASTING, CRYOTHERAPY, AND OTHER NEW TECHNIQUES PLAY IMPORTANT ROLES IN ANTI-AGING SCIENCE.

In the effort to reduce aging, scientific discoveries are constantly unveiling new ways with promising outcomes. **Fasting, cryotherapy**, and other novel therapies attempt to improve longevity, cellular repair, and general vitality.

1. Fasting: Caloric restriction and intermittent fasting

Fasting, particularly **intermittent fasting (IF)** and **calorie restriction,** is widely recognized as one of the most effective treatments for reducing the aging process. These strategies are based on the premise that lowering calorie intake or restricting meal times triggers a variety of biological pathways that enhance health and longevity.

• **Caloric Restriction (CR):** Research from the 1930s suggests that limiting calorie intake by 20–40% while maintaining nutrient intake will lengthen lifespans in animals like mice, rats, and monkeys. The reduction in calories activates metabolic pathways that promote **cellular repair**, **reduce inflammation**, and **lower oxidative stress**, all of which are important variables in aging.

• **Intermittent fasting (IF)** entails alternating between eating and fasting, such as 16/8 (fasting for 16 hours and eating for 8) or 5:2 (five days of normal eating and two days of severe calorie restriction). IF promotes **autophagy**, a process in which the body eliminates damaged cells and regenerates new ones, which contributes to slower aging and a lower risk of diseases such as Alzheimer's, heart disease, and cancer.

For example, Dr. Valter Longo's research on the **Fasting Mimicking Diet (FMD)**, which allows people to gain the benefits of fasting while still eating, has demonstrated that it improves cellular regeneration and lowers aging and disease indicators.

2. Cryotherapy: The Power of Cold Exposure

Cryotherapy, or exposing the body to extremely cold temperatures for a brief period of time (usually -150°C to -200°C for 2-3 minutes), is becoming increasingly popular as a rehabilitation and anti-aging method. Advocates of cryotherapy believe that it offers several health benefits, including faster recovery, less inflammation, and improved metabolic efficiency.

- **Cellular Stress Response**: The cold induces a stress reaction in the body, generating **endorphins** and increasing blood flow. Cold exposure also boosts the creation of **brown fat** (a type of fat that burns energy) and promotes **mitochondrial function,** which is critical for slowing the aging process.

• **Inflammation and Recovery:** Cryotherapy can help reduce **inflammation and swelling** by restricting blood vessels. This is especially useful for athletes and elderly persons who want to keep their muscles and joints healthy.

For example, athletes like LeBron James and celebrities like Tony Robbins have adopted cryotherapy as part of their wellness and anti-aging routines, despite the fact that its long-term effects on aging are still being explored.

3. Advanced Stem Cell Therapy

Stem cell therapy is one of the most promising developments in anti-aging research. Researchers are investigating ways to regenerate tissues, repair damaged organs, and potentially reverse the effects of aging using

mesenchymal stem cells (MSCs), which can develop into many types of cells.

- **Regenerative Power**: Stem cells have the ability to regenerate damaged tissues, including cartilage in joints, heart muscles, and neurons in the brain. Our bodies' natural stem cell reserves dwindle with age, resulting in slower recovery and greater vulnerability to age-related illnesses. Supplementing the body with stem cells could be a breakthrough method to combat these effects.

- **Tissue Rejuvenation**: Recent research suggests that stem cells can regenerate skin, boost hair regeneration, and heal degenerative disorders, leading to increased longevity and quality of life.

For example, researchers are experimenting with infusing stem cells into aging organs to reverse the effects of age. Clinics all over the world now provide stem cell treatments as part of anti-aging programs, albeit these treatments are still pricey and under clinical evaluation.

Action Step: Supplement Guide for Anti-Aging

To assist readers in developing a supplement routine that supports graceful aging, here is a complete guide that contains crucial nutrients, dosages, and when they may be effective. These supplements should enhance, rather than replace, a well-balanced diet and a healthy lifestyle. Always consult a healthcare expert before incorporating new supplements into your routine, especially if you have underlying health concerns or are using drugs.

1. Vitamin D

• **Why Take It:** It promotes bone density, immunological function, and muscle health, which are important as we age. Deficiency is frequent in older persons due to a lack of sun exposure.

• **Recommended daily dosage:** 1,000-2,000 IU, based on baseline blood levels and locale.

• **When to Add:** Consider adding vitamin D if you live in a place with minimal sunlight, especially during the winter months, or spend a lot of time indoors.

2. Omega-3 Fatty Acids (EPA and DHA)

• **Why Take It**: Omega-3s promote heart health and brain function and reduce inflammation, which is associated with age-related disorders.

• **Recommended Dosage**: 1,000-2,000 mg of EPA and DHA combined.

• **When to Add**: Consider taking an omega-3 supplement for cardiovascular and cognitive health if you don't consume enough oily fish (e.g., salmon or mackerel).

3. Resveratrol

• **Why Take It:** A polyphenol with anti-aging qualities activates SIRT1 genes and mimics the benefits of calorie restriction.

- **Recommended dosage:** 150 to 500 mg daily. Higher doses are frequently utilized in clinical research, although further research is required to determine long-term safety.

- **When to Add:** Resveratrol can provide cellular effects akin to calorie restriction without limiting food intake.

4. Coenzyme Q-10 (CoQ10)

- **Why Take It:** Boosts energy production, especially in the heart and muscles, and may alleviate weariness in older persons.

- **Recommended dosage:** 100-300 mg per day with a fat-rich meal for optimal absorption.

- **When to Add**: CoQ10 is especially useful if you are on statin medications, which can deplete natural levels of this coenzyme, or if you experience fatigue and low energy.

5. NAD+ precursors (NR or NMN)

• **Why Take It:** NAD+ promotes cellular repair, mitochondrial health, and DNA repair. NAD+ levels diminish with age, which has been linked to accelerated aging.

• **The recommended daily dose** is 250-500 mg of nicotinamide riboside (NR) or nicotinamide mononucleotide.

• **When to Add:** NAD+ boosters may benefit anyone over 40 seeking cellular energy support or improved mitochondrial health.

6. Collagen

• **Why Take It:** Promotes skin elasticity, joint health, and muscle mass. Collagen production naturally decreases with age, resulting in wrinkles and joint stiffness.

•**Recommended Dosage**: Take 5 to 10 grams of collagen peptides per day.

• **When to Add**: Consider adding collagen if experiencing skin aging, joint stiffness, or loss of muscular mass. It's especially useful if you're physically active or over 50.

7. Magnesium

• **Why Take It:** Promotes muscle relaxation, bone health, and sleep quality. Magnesium deficits can exacerbate sleep issues and raise the risk of osteoporosis.

• **Recommended dosage:** 300-400 mg daily, with magnesium glycinate or citrate for improved absorption.

• **When to Add**: Magnesium supplementation can enhance sleep, muscle cramping, and anxiety, leading to better overall well-being.

8. Probiotics

• **Why Take It**: Gut health improves immunity, digestion, and overall health. Probiotics help maintain a healthy balance of intestinal bacteria, which can deteriorate with age.

- **Recommended dosage:** ranges from 1 to 10 billion CFU per day, according to strain and health needs.

- **When to Add**: Add a high-quality probiotic to restore gut health if experiencing digestive difficulties, immunological dysfunction, or recent antibiotic use.

Incorporating the correct supplements into your daily routine can help with crucial aspects of aging, such as bone and heart health, cognitive function, and cell repair. However, remember that supplements work best when accompanied by a nutrient-dense diet, frequent exercise, and adequate sleep. By monitoring your body's response and making modifications as needed, you can fine-tune your supplement intake to support a longer, healthier lifestyle.

4. NAD+ therapy promotes cellular energy and repair.

NAD+ (Nicotinamide Adenine Dinucleotide) is a coenzyme involved in **cellular metabolism** and **DNA repair**. As we age, our NAD+ levels fall, resulting in decreased energy production and worse cellular repair mechanisms. This hastens aging.

• **Boosting NAD+**: Supplementing with NAD+ precursors, such as **nicotinamide riboside (NR)** or **nicotinamide mononucleotide (NMN)**, is thought to restore these levels, leading to improved mitochondrial function, enhanced energy production, and activation of **sirtuins**—proteins associated with aging and longevity.

• **Longevity Potential:** Animal studies suggest that increasing NAD+ levels can improve physical health and extend longevity. NAD+ supplements are now widely available and employed in anti-aging regimens to rejuvenate cells.

For example, researchers such as Dr. David Sinclair have popularized NAD+ therapy, arguing that it can increase longevity and reverse parts of biological aging in mice. Human studies are underway, and preliminary results indicate increased physical performance and cellular health.

Where Does Cutting-Edge Anti-Aging Science Stand?

The science of aging is rapidly evolving, with fasting, cryotherapy, stem cell therapy, and NAD+ boosting at the forefront of research and innovation. While many of these strategies appear promising, it is crucial to highlight that much of the science is still growing, particularly in long-term human trials. What is evident, however, is that a holistic approach—combining these modern medicines with lifestyle adjustments such as nutrition, exercise, and mental health practices—is the most effective way to age gracefully and sustain energy in later life.

Chapter 10

The Strength of Purpose and Positivity in Aging

Finding Meaning in Every Stage of Life: How a Sense of Purpose Increases Longevity and Happiness

One of the most fundamental, yet frequently underestimated, components of healthy aging is the importance of **purpose** and **positivity** in longevity. Numerous studies have shown that having a sense of purpose, whether through employment, hobbies, relationships, or community activity, can have a substantial impact on not just how long but also how well we live. Indeed, studies demonstrate that older persons who have a strong sense of purpose are less likely to experience cognitive decline, cardiovascular disease, and even death.

The Science of Purpose and Longevity

The scientific evidence for the health benefits of living a purposeful life is growing. According to a 2014 study published in The Lancet, those who have a clear sense of purpose live longer lives than those who do not. Similarly, the Okinawa Centenarian Study, which looked at some of the world's oldest people, attributed much of their longevity to a concept known as **"ikigai,"** or a "reason for being." Okinawans play an active role in their communities and find meaning in everything they do, from gardening to caring for grandchildren. This sense of responsibility and connection, they believe, is just as important as any physical fitness plan.

Why Purpose Improves Health and Longevity.

But why does purpose have such a strong influence on our health? There are a number of physiological and psychological causes behind this:

1. Stress Reduction: Having a clear sense of purpose lowers cortisol levels, a stress hormone associated with premature aging and a variety of age-related illnesses. When people believe that their lives have value, they are better prepared to deal with stress and avoid its negative consequences on the heart, brain, and immune system.

2. Motivation to Stay Active: A feeling of purpose can help people sustain healthy behaviors, including regular physical activity, healthy food, and social involvement. When we believe we are contributing to something bigger than ourselves, we are more willing to care for our physical bodies in order to continue performing that role.

3. **Social Connections:** Purpose is typically associated with relationships, whether familial, communal, or spiritual. Maintaining social relationships has been demonstrated to reduce the incidence of depression, cognitive decline, and chronic illnesses, making it an important aspect in aging healthily.

4. **Mental Stimulation:** Performing meaningful things keeps the brain busy. Mental stimulation is critical to preventing cognitive decline and disorders such as **Alzheimer's.** Volunteering, mentoring, and engaging in

artistic pursuits are all examples of purposeful activities that challenge the mind and increase neuroplasticity—the brain's ability to develop new connections and pathways.

Purpose Across Life Stages.

Purpose appears differently at various phases of life. For younger people, purpose may be related to job ambitions, starting a family, or academic achievements. These aspirations may change as we get older, but the urge for meaning remains. In subsequent years, purpose might be found in:

• **Mentorship:** Older persons can pass on expertise to future generations through family or community involvement.

• **Creative pursuits**, such as art, writing, and hobbies, can provide a deep sense of fulfillment.

• **Community Engagement:** Volunteering, activism, or joining in local groups can help you stay socially connected and positively impact others.

• **Spirituality:** For many, faith and spirituality provide a sense of purpose, especially during life's closing chapters. This may include religious practices, meditation, or personal reflection.

The tremendous impact of purpose in mental health is not a novel concept. Psychologist Viktor Frankl, a Holocaust survivor and author of Man's Search for Meaning, created logotherapy, a type of existential therapy based on the notion that our major motivation in life is not pleasure, but the discovery and pursuit of what we personally find significant. Frankl claimed that finding meaning, even in the most terrible circumstances, enabled people to overcome pain and live completely.

In the context of aging, Frankl's lessons remind us that a feeling of purpose does not fade with time but rather changes. Even as physical capabilities deteriorate, the ability to discover meaning remains.

A POSITIVE OUTLOOK IS PART OF THE EQUATION

Positive attitudes also influence how we age. According to research, older persons who have a positive attitude toward aging live an average of **7.5 years longer** than those who have a negative attitude. A good mindset affects not only mental health but also how the body deals with stress, inflammation, and even how the immune system works.

A feeling of purpose combined with a good attitude can be the perfect combination for a long, healthy, and fulfilled life. It is not enough to simply add years to your life; you must also add vitality to your years. Daily purpose gives us something to strive for, care about, and contribute. That is one of the most effective anti-aging tools at our disposal.

The Psychology of Aging Well: How a Positive Outlook and Emotional Resiliency Contribute to Longevity

Aging is unavoidable, but how we age is determined by a variety of factors, many of which we can influence. Research in psychology and gerontology has revealed that emotional well-being and resilience are essential for healthy aging. These features, while often overlooked in talks about health and longevity, have far-reaching implications for both physical and cognitive health as we age. An optimistic view on life and the ability to deal with hardship not only improve our quality of life but can also extend it.

Positive outlook and longevity

A positive perspective entails more than simply having an optimistic demeanor. It is a manner of interpreting life's circumstances that enables people to find purpose and hope, even when faced with adversity. This approach has been related to better aging for a variety of reasons.

1. Psychological Resilience to Stress

Stress is an unavoidable aspect of life, yet our reactions to it can differ dramatically. Older persons with a positive outlook are better able to deal with stress. A 2004 study in the Journal of Personality and Social Psychology discovered that optimism was linked to lower stress levels and healthier cortisol responses. Chronic stress is known to promote biological aging by shortening telomeres, which are protective caps on the ends of our chromosomes that deteriorate over time. A good attitude helps lessen this effect.

Consider the situation of centenarians, who live to be 100 or older. According to research, these people share psychological characteristics such as optimism, low neuroticism, and the ability to adjust to life's adversities.

Their tolerance to stress plays a significant part in their longer lifespans.

2. Impact on immune function

There is a strong link between our mental state and immunological function. According to research, positive emotions can boost the immune system, whereas persistent negative emotions like anger, depression, or worry suppress it. For example, Sheldon Cohen of Carnegie Mellon University discovered that persons who feel positive emotions such as joy and satisfaction are less prone to contract colds and other infectious diseases. This is especially important as we become older because our immune systems typically weaken. Older folks who have a positive attitude may experience fewer diseases and recover faster when they do get sick.

3. Improved health habits

A cheerful mindset can also help you live longer by encouraging you to adopt healthier habits. People with a positive outlook are more likely to engage in health-promoting activities such as exercise, consuming a balanced diet, and following medical advice. A big longitudinal study from Harvard discovered that optimism was linked to a longer lifetime, with a considerable chunk of this benefit mediated by better behaviors. One example is the well-known Nun Study, which looked into the lives of over 700 nuns, focusing on their writing samples as young women and subsequent life outcomes. Nuns who displayed more pleasant feelings in their teens lived substantially longer than those who were more pessimistic. Importantly, the nuns lived in similar environmental settings, implying that their thinking had a significant impact on their health.

Emotional Resilience and Aging

Emotional resilience is the ability to recover from hardship, stress, and traumatic events. As we get older, we face more physical and social challenges, such as decreasing health, the death of loved ones, or even retirement, which can lead to a loss of identity and purpose. How we handle these issues greatly affects our aging.

1. Cognitive function and emotional resilience

People who are emotionally resilient tend to have better cognitive outcomes in old age. The capacity to handle stress and remain calm under pressure has been related to a lower risk of cognitive decline and diseases such as Alzheimer's. This is because prolonged stress causes inflammation and oxidative stress, both of which can harm brain cells over time. Emotional resilience guards against this.

Holocaust survivors provide an eye-opening example of perseverance in the face of enormous trauma. Many survivors maintain excellent cognitive function and mental health well into old age. Their ability to cope with trauma—via social support, finding meaning in their experiences, and remaining hopeful—enabled them to reduce the long-term impacts of stress on their brains.

2. Creating Social Support Networks

Emotionally resilient people are also more likely to form and maintain robust social support networks, which are essential for healthy aging. Social involvement keeps the mind active and prevents emotions of loneliness, which are a major risk factor for cognitive decline and premature death. In fact, a 2015 meta-analysis in Perspectives on Psychological Science discovered that loneliness increased the chance of premature death by 26%, making it a more significant risk factor than obesity.

Consider Mediterranean regions noted for longevity, such as Sardinia in Italy and Ikaria in Greece. People in these places live a long life, thanks in part to their plant-based diets and strong communal bonds. Elderly individuals remain active, socially involved, and appreciated in their families and communities, which improves their emotional well-being and resilience.

Practical Steps for Developing a Positive Outlook and Emotional Resilience

While some people are innately more optimistic or resilient, these qualities can be developed through deliberate practice.

1. Gratitude Practice: Keeping a gratitude notebook or constantly reflecting on what one is grateful for might help shift one's attention from the negative to the good parts of life. According to research, people who practice gratitude report having a better mood, less stress, and even better sleep.

2. Mindfulness and meditation: Mindfulness-based stress reduction (MBSR) programs have been demonstrated to lower stress, improve emotional resilience, and even increase longevity. Older folks can lessen their anxiety and rumination by focusing on the present moment and accepting it without judgment.

3. Cognitive Behavioral Therapy (CBT): CBT has been shown to be beneficial in retraining negative thought processes in persons suffering from persistent negativity or emotional difficulties. It enables people to notice and question skewed thinking, as well as replace it with more balanced and constructive views.

4. Social Connections: Participating in community events, volunteering, or simply maintaining friendships can boost emotional resilience. Older persons who remain socially active have a lower risk of depression and anxiety and live longer lives.

5. Physical Activity: Exercise is essential for both physical and mental health. Physical activity lowers stress, improves mood, and promotes neuroplasticity— the brain's ability to change and rearrange itself, which is essential for sustaining cognitive function in old age.

Mind-Body Connection in Aging

The psychology of aging emphasizes the profound relationship between the mind and body. An optimistic attitude and emotional resilience are more than just desirable personality traits; they are important predictors of longevity. Individuals who cultivate these qualities can protect themselves from aging-related pressures, maintain physical and cognitive health, and ultimately live a longer, better life.

The scientific lesson is clear: aging is about how we live our lives rather than how many years we have. Those who can create emotional resilience and keep a positive outlook are more likely to not only live longer but also thrive in their older years. The key to longevity, it turns out, is as much mental as physical.

Action Step: A Guide to Finding Purpose in Your Daily Life and Setting Long-Term Goals, Regardless of Age

Purpose provides your life meaning, direction, and fulfillment. Purpose is not simply a concept for the young or those pursuing careers; it is an essential component of emotional well-being and longevity at all stages of life. Research regularly shows that having a sense of purpose is linked to a longer life, improved health outcomes, and increased pleasure. However, finding meaning and defining long-term goals can be difficult, especially when we get older, go through life transitions, or confront hardships.

Whether you're 25 or 85, having a cause to get up in the morning can improve your quality of life. Let us break this down into simple stages to help you uncover your purpose in life and develop meaningful goals for the future.

1. Reflect on your core values and beliefs.

Understanding yourself is the first step in discovering your mission. What are you deeply concerned about? Which values guide your decisions, and how do you want to help? These questions can function as a compass.

Action Step

• **List your core values:** Spend 10 to 15 minutes writing down what matters most to you. This could involve family, creativity, helping others, education, health, spirituality, or environmental stewardship.

• **Evaluate Current Alignment:** Check if your daily behaviors correspond with these values. If not, consider how you may change your routine to better reflect your values.

If you enjoy studying but haven't had the opportunity to explore new topics, consider taking a class, reading a book, or attending a local lecture. If family is a priority, create time for meaningful interactions, whether through daily phone conversations or a weekly meeting.

2. Identify your strengths and interests

Purpose frequently develops when you do activities you enjoy and excel at. Your hobbies, skills, and interests can help you identify where your abilities cross with your sense of purpose.

Action Step

• **Strengths Inventory:** Take stock of your natural strengths and skills. Are you a good listener? Do you excel at organizing? Are you artistic or musically inclined? Write these down.

- **Interest Exploration:** Make a list of activities that genuinely engage you. Consider hobbies you've enjoyed, topics you like to read about, or areas of life where you naturally feel "in the zone."

Once you've identified your strengths and hobbies, think about how you may incorporate more of them into your everyday routine or make goals to further develop them. For example, if you enjoy teaching and mentoring, consider volunteering to tutor or coach others.

3. Engage in mindfulness and self-reflection.

Sometimes we lose sight of our purpose because we are preoccupied with the daily grind or uncomfortable emotions. Cultivating mindfulness allows us to step back, calm the noise, and reconnect with what is truly important.

Action Step

- **Daily Mindfulness Practice:** Set aside 10 to 15 minutes per day to practice mindfulness or meditation. This does not have to be complicated; simply concentrate on your breath or take a mindful walk, paying attention to the sensations of your steps and surroundings.

- **Journal for Clarity:** Reflect on what makes you feel alive. Consider experiences where you were genuinely fulfilled. What happened throughout those moments? How can you reproduce or incorporate parts of those experiences into your current life?

Over time, mindfulness and introspection can show patterns in what provides you joy and fulfillment, allowing you to find potential paths for meaning.

4. Break down the purpose into small, achievable goals.

Purpose does not need to be a great, life-changing mission. It can be discovered in tiny, ordinary actions that contribute to a meaningful life. Instead of looking for a single overarching purpose, consider it a collection of important goals, both short- and long-term.

Action Step

• **Set SMART goals** (Specific, Measurable, Achievable, Relevant, and Time-bound). Begin by setting a small, attainable objective that is consistent with your values and interests. For example, if you want to stay healthy, set a goal of walking for 30 minutes three times a week.

• **Break down long-term goals into manageable milestones,** such as starting a new career or learning a new skill. For example, if you want to write a book, establish a goal of 500 words every day. This makes enormous goals more manageable.

Setting smaller goals allows you to retain momentum and enjoy tiny wins, which will keep you motivated in the long run.

5. Embrace change and flexibility.

Purpose and goals might shift throughout time. What motivates you in your 30s may not be the same as what makes you satisfied in your 60s or later. The trick is to be adaptive and open to changing interests and situations.

Action Step

• **Regularly review and revise your goals** to ensure they correspond with your sense of purpose. It is absolutely acceptable to change directions if new interests or opportunities arise.

• **Embrace New Roles:** Life transitions, such as retirement, empty nesting, or health changes, can cause a loss of identity and purpose. Reframe these experiences as chances for growth. For example, retirees may find fulfillment in teaching younger generations, traveling, or revisiting long-forgotten interests.

6. Contribute to something bigger than yourself.

Contributing to others or a cause larger than oneself is one of the most potent sources of purpose. According to research, persons who engage in prosocial conduct, such as volunteering, assisting others, or giving back to their communities, have a stronger sense of purpose and fulfillment.

Action Step

• **Volunteer for a Cause You Care About:** Volunteering at a local shelter, tutoring youngsters, or fighting for environmental sustainability can provide a strong sense of purpose.

• **Random Acts of Kindness:** Small acts of kindness, such as helping a neighbor or lending a listening ear, can bring significance to your day and boost your sense of purpose.

7. Foster social connections.

Strong social ties are essential components of a fulfilling life. Engaging with others provides us with a sense of belonging and reminds us that we are part of a broader community.

Action Step

• **Nurture Existing Relationships:** Invest time and energy into maintaining strong relationships with family, friends, and colleagues. Set a goal of reaching out on a regular basis, whether by phone calls, text messages, or in-person visits.

• **Seek New Connections:** Join a local club, group, or organization to connect with others who share your interests. Building new social relationships can help you rediscover your sense of purpose.

8. Be open to learning and development.

Purpose is not static; it changes as we do. Stay curious and open to learning new things throughout your life. Continuing to learn new skills and knowledge can be energizing and provide a sense of achievement.

Action Step

• **Take a Class or Learn a New Skill:** It's never too late to learn. Painting, computing, cooking, or learning a new language are all examples of new experiences that can provide delight and help you discover a new sense of purpose.

• **Read and Stay Informed:** Stay informed by reading books, articles, or podcasts about topics you're interested in. Lifelong learning keeps you adaptive and open to new opportunities.

9. Celebrate progress and achievements.

Recognizing your accomplishments, no matter how minor, emphasizes the value of your work and keeps you motivated.

Action Step

• **Establish a Gratitude Ritual:** At the end of each day, reflect on your accomplishments, gratitudes, and progress towards your goals. This straightforward activity increases your sense of purpose by emphasizing the importance of your daily tasks.

Developing Purpose as a Lifelong Process

Finding meaning and developing long-term goals is a continual process. No matter your age, establishing purpose in daily life entails recognizing your underlying values, participating in meaningful activities, remaining adaptable in the face of life's changes, and contributing to something bigger than yourself. By taking tiny, conscious steps every day, you may create a meaningful life and continue to establish and achieve goals that offer you fulfillment, happiness, and longevity.

Chapter 11

Real-Life Success Stories.

Inspirational Case Studies: Exceptional Results from Applying the Principles of Purpose and Longevity

Nothing conveys the transformative power of purpose, resilience, and positive thinking like real-life instances of people who have adopted these ideas and experienced the benefits. The following stories include people from various walks of life, ages, and backgrounds who have discovered meaning, perseverance, and purpose in their journeys. These examples demonstrate how having an optimistic attitude, adopting important goals, and adapting to life's challenges can lead to satisfying and thriving lives, regardless of age or condition.

1. John's Story: Purpose and Reinvention in Retirement

John has always identified himself through his career. As a successful attorney, his life was filled with deadlines, courtroom appearances, and lengthy office hours. When

John retired at age 65, he was at a loss. The rituals and structure that had directed his life for decades vanished, leaving him feeling empty and purposeless. He became depressed, unsure what to do with his newfound independence.

Turning Point: Discovering the Purpose in Mentoring

John realized he needed to regain control of his life. After considerable thought, he recognized that mentoring younger lawyers had always been the most enjoyable component of his employment. He decided to contact the local law schools and offer his services as a volunteer mentor.

Within months, John had reconnected to his feeling of purpose. He got actively involved in his community, guiding legal students through their early careers. When his confidence returned, he found teaching and coaching as rewarding—if not more so—than court. John's health improved, and his despair subsided.

John now wakes up every day with a purpose, eager to continue guiding the next generation of attorneys. In retirement, John discovered contentment and happiness by recreating himself and focusing on his abilities and interests.

2. Maria's Story: Resilience Following Loss

Maria, a 70-year-old widow, experienced indescribable anguish when her husband of 45 years died. Maria was depressed, lonely, and lost for months. She had always been a caregiver, first for her children and later for her husband while he was unwell. After his death, she felt she no longer had a part to play and questioned her life's purpose.

Turning Point: Discovering Meaning in Helping Others

Maria read about a local hospice program looking for volunteers to provide companionship to terminally ill patients. She sparked an interest and wanted to try it. While it was tough at first, Maria soon found consolation in helping others who were going through similar experiences. The thanks she got from patients and their families renewed her sense of purpose.

Maria now volunteers three days a week at the hospice, guiding people through the end-of-life process with compassion and grace. Her resilience in the face of loss has not only aided her healing but has also enabled her to discover great purpose in her daily life. Maria frequently states that the work she does today gives her more fulfillment than she ever dreamed of after her husband's death.

3. Daniel's Story: Getting Over Chronic Illness with a Positive Outlook

Daniel was diagnosed with a chronic autoimmune illness in his mid-fifties. The illness greatly restricted his movement, resulting in joint pain, weariness, and difficulties doing daily duties. Daniel struggled to adjust to his new limits, falling into a spiral of negativity and self-pity. His health began to worsen more as melancholy and anxiety set in.

Turning Point: Changing Perspective and Establishing Health Goals

A meeting with his doctor served as the catalyst for transformation. His doctor highlighted the importance of mindset in managing chronic illness, advising Daniel to focus on what he could accomplish rather than what he couldn't. Daniel began practicing gratitude and mindfulness on a daily basis, incorporating modest, positive modifications into his routine.

He also established attainable fitness goals, such as 15 minutes of light stretching every morning, followed by gentle walking. Daniel noted that his symptoms gradually stabilized, and his mental attitude improved substantially. Inspired by his improvement, he joined a local chronic disease support group, where he discovered kinship and strength from others going through similar experiences.

Today, Daniel candidly discusses the importance of a positive mindset in managing chronic illness. Though his disease persists, Daniel claims his quality of life has much improved. His mental strength has not only helped him manage his symptoms, but it has also revived his enthusiasm for life. He attributes his longevity and well-being to a small but fundamental alteration in his mindset.

4. Eleanor's Story: Finding Purpose After Retirement

Eleanor was a career-oriented woman who spent decades establishing a thriving business consultancy. When she retired at 68, she rapidly became bored. She had always thrived in high-energy settings and felt adrift without the continual stimulation and difficulties of her job. Like many retirees, she struggled to adjust to a slower pace of life.

Turning Point: Learning to Focus on New Goals

Eleanor learned that just because she was out of business did not mean she had nothing to contribute. Reflecting on what she enjoyed most about her job, she discovered her true passion was assisting others in growing their businesses and improving their leadership skills. She decided to transform her interest into a part-time consulting service for small business owners in her area.

Eleanor felt energized after setting new, smaller goals, such as assisting one new business each month. She also set a long-term goal of authoring a book on leadership, leveraging her years of experience to help the next generation of business owners. Eleanor's purpose and drive have kept her physically and mentally active, and she feels more involved than ever. She now sees retirement not as the end of her career but as an opportunity to apply her skills to something as important.

5. Kenji's Story: Finding Fulfillment Through Community Service

Kenji, 62, had spent the majority of his life working in a high-pressure business setting. When his company shrank and Kenji lost his job, he experienced an identity crisis. He felt detached from his neighborhood and tried to find ways to spend his time. For the first time, he questioned what made his life meaningful outside of work.

Turning Point: Volunteering for a Local Cause

Kenji chose to help at a local food bank. At first, he saw it as a method to keep himself busy, but he quickly discovered that giving back to his community provided him with deep happiness. Interacting with volunteers and assisting families in need offered Kenji a new sense of purpose. He realized that his former job, while financially gratifying, did not completely fulfill him.

Volunteering became a regular occurrence, and Kenji began organizing food drives and fundraising for local charity. Over time, his community involvement allowed him to reclaim his sense of identity and self-worth. Kenji now sees his post-career existence as an opportunity to positively impact the lives of others.

6. Lillian's Story: Embracing a Second Career After 60

Lillian had always enjoyed painting but had never taken it seriously. She had worked as a nurse for many years, which she found fulfilling but physically and emotionally demanding. After retiring at the age of 60, Lillian decided to take a chance and enroll in art lessons at a nearby community center.

Turning Point: Setting Creative Goals and Building Confidence

Though cautious at first, Lillian made a personal goal of creating and exhibiting at least five of her paintings in a local art show within a year. She worked hard to hone her talents and started sharing her work with friends and family, who encouraged her to continue.

By the age of 65, Lillian had held her first solo show, and her work was well received. She learned that pursuing her interest not only kept her mind and body active but also led to new friendships and opportunities. Painting had given her life new meaning, and she now refers to herself as a "late-blooming artist." Today, Lillian continues to paint and has even started teaching art to seniors, assisting them in discovering their own creative potential.

The Power of Purpose in Action.

These stories demonstrate the tremendous transformation that occurs when people take conscious measures to discover their purpose and set meaningful goals. Whether it was suffering personal loss, adjusting to retirement, or managing chronic illness, each person featured here found their inner strength, reinvented their purpose, and made concrete steps toward a more rewarding life. Their adventures emphasize the universal fact that purpose is not age-bound and that we can all find and redefine meaning, regardless of our circumstances.

These people demonstrate that by aligning our behaviors with our beliefs, setting attainable goals, and remaining adaptable in the face of change, we can live rich, meaningful lives full of purpose—even as we age.

INTERVIEWS WITH EXPERTS: INCREASING CREDIBILITY WITH QUOTES FROM DOCTORS, RESEARCHERS, AND NUTRITIONISTS

To reinforce the concepts of healthy aging, such as maintaining a happy outlook, cultivating emotional resilience, and discovering purpose, we will seek the advice of specialists in medicine, psychology, and nutrition. Their findings not only lend scientific support to these notions but also provide practical guidance for anyone wishing to improve their health and longevity. Here are some professional viewpoints on the secrets to having a long, healthy, and fulfilling life.

Dr. Sarah Mitchell is a geriatrician and longevity expert

Dr. Sarah Mitchell has spent more than 20 years researching the elements that influence healthy aging, both physically and emotionally. Her research on healthy aging highlights the importance of emotional well-being and maintaining a positive attitude.

Those who see aging as a time of growth and opportunity tend to live longer, healthier lives. A positive outlook not only makes you feel better—it also has profound effects on physical health. Studies show that optimism is linked to lower levels of inflammation, a lower risk of cardiovascular disease, and even a stronger immune system. Aging well is about more than just avoiding disease.

Dr. Mitchell emphasizes the necessity of emotional resilience in dealing with life's unavoidable adversities.

"Emotional resilience—the ability to bounce back from adversity—is one of the most critical traits for healthy aging. I often tell my patients that resilience is like a muscle; the more you use it, the stronger it becomes. Practices like mindfulness, gratitude, and staying socially connected are key ways to build and maintain emotional resilience.

Dr. Martin Kleinman is a clinical psychologist and aging researcher.

Dr. Martin Kleinman's research focuses on the psychological aspects of aging, specifically how purpose and goal-setting affect mental well-being as we age. He has thoroughly researched the advantages of purpose-driven living for elders.

"Purpose is a crucial component of psychological well-being. It's not just about having a career or raising a family—it's about feeling that your life has meaning, no matter your age or circumstances. Research shows that older adults with a strong sense of purpose are less likely to suffer from depression, anxiety, and even cognitive decline. They're also more likely to engage in healthy behaviors, like exercising regularly, eating well, and staying socially active."

Dr. Kleinman frequently tells his clients to remain open to new opportunities, regardless of their age.

"There's a common misconception that finding purpose is something only for young people or those in the middle of their careers. But I've seen firsthand that purpose evolves with time. In fact, many people find deeper meaning later in life, whether it's through community service, artistic expression, or mentoring others. The key is to remain curious and engaged, always looking for new ways to contribute to the world around you."

Dr. Fiona Richardson, Nutritionist and Aging Specialist

Dr. Fiona Richardson is a prominent nutritionist whose study focuses on the relationship between diet and longevity. She believes that what we eat is crucial to not only prolonging our lives but also sustaining mental and physical energy as we age.

"The link between nutrition and longevity is undeniable. A diet rich in whole foods—fruits, vegetables, whole grains, nuts, and lean proteins—provides the body with the nutrients it needs to fight inflammation, maintain cognitive function, and reduce the risk of chronic diseases like heart disease, diabetes, and cancer. But beyond physical health, nutrition also influences mental health. Omega-3 fatty acids, found in fish like salmon, are essential for the brain.

Dr. Richardson urges her clients to think of food as more than just sustenance; it's also a form of self-care and connection.

"One of the most powerful things I emphasize is that food can be a source of joy and connection. Sharing meals with loved ones, preparing healthy foods together, or growing your own produce fosters emotional well-being and helps build social connections, which are essential for aging well. The experience of nourishing your body and spirit is more than the nutrients."

Dr. Jonathan Williams is a cardiologist and longevity researcher.

As a cardiologist, Dr. Jonathan Williams studies the link between heart health and lifespan. His research focuses on how positive emotional health, regular exercise, and a heart-healthy diet can significantly increase lifespan.

"When we talk about heart health, we're really talking about total health. The heart is incredibly sensitive to our emotional and psychological state. Chronic stress, anxiety, and depression can all contribute to higher blood pressure, heart disease, and other cardiovascular issues. On the flip side, practicing emotional resilience and cultivating positive relationships can lower stress hormones like cortisol, which directly benefits heart health."

Dr. Williams is a strong supporter of regular physical activity, emphasizing that it does not have to be strenuous to have a significant difference.

"You don't need to run marathons to keep your heart healthy—though if that's your passion, go for it! The key is to stay active in ways that you enjoy. Whether it's walking, gardening, swimming, or yoga, physical movement is essential for maintaining both cardiovascular health and emotional well-being. Regular exercise has been shown to reduce the risk of heart disease, improve mood, and even boost cognitive function as we age."

Dr. Emily Thompson, cognitive neuroscientist

Dr. Emily Thompson focuses on the study of cognitive decline and brain health in older persons. Her research highlights the role of mental stimulation and social involvement in avoiding dementia and Alzheimer's disease.

"The brain, like the body, thrives on use. Cognitive decline is not an inevitable part of aging; it is often the result of disuse. Keeping the brain active through challenging tasks—whether it's learning a new language, playing a musical instrument, or solving puzzles—can help preserve cognitive function well into old age. Social interaction is equally important. People who maintain strong social networks and engage in regular conversations are less likely to experience

Dr. Thompson emphasizes the importance of emotional health in preserving cognitive sharpness.

"There's a growing body of evidence that suggests a direct link between emotional health and cognitive function. Stress, anxiety, and depression are all risk factors for cognitive decline, while positive emotional experiences—like laughter, social interaction, and practicing gratitude—are protective. Simply put, what's beneficial for your mind and heart is also beneficial for your brain."

Dr. Michael Gupta is a psychologist and mindfulness expert

Dr. Michael Gupta has spent his career researching how mindfulness and emotional regulation lead to a long and fulfilled life. He has vast experience working with older persons to build strategies that promote emotional resilience and well-being.

"Mindfulness is a powerful tool for aging well. It teaches people to be present, to accept life as it is, and to reduce the stress and anxiety that often come with aging. When people practice mindfulness, they're able to cultivate a sense of peace and contentment, even in the face of physical or emotional challenges. The research is clear—mindfulness can lower blood pressure, improve sleep, reduce chronic pain, and boost mood."

Dr. Gupta frequently adds thankfulness techniques into his work with clients.

I encourage people of all ages to keep a gratitude journal or simply take a few moments each day to reflect on the positive things in their lives. Focusing on what we're grateful for—whether it's the beauty of nature, the kindness of a friend, or a cherished memory—brings us into the present moment and lifts our spirits. This emotional shift can have long-term effects on both mental and physical health.

Expert endorsements and actionable insights.

These experts' insights—ranging from psychology and nutrition to cardiology and cognitive neuroscience—send a clear message: aging properly is a comprehensive process. Individuals can add years to their lives and life to their years by having a happy outlook, creating goals that correspond with personal values, remaining physically active, and fostering emotional and social well-being.

These expert viewpoints give the scientific basis for the practices described in previous chapters. They remind us that, while aging is unavoidable, the way we age is mainly under our control. With the correct mindset, lifestyle choices, and emotional resiliency, we can thrive at any age.

Conclusion

Bringing It All Together

Aging is an unavoidable part of life, yet as we've seen throughout this book, how we age is mainly under our control. Each chapter has provided essential insights and specific methods to help you control your aging process, shifting it from a source of anxiety to an opportunity for development, vitality, and purpose. To reflect on and apply the principles you've learned, let's review each chapter's key takeaways.

Chapter One: Understanding the Aging Process

We began by looking at the biological mechanisms of aging, such as telomere shortening and cellular senescence, which lead our bodies to degrade over time. However, we also investigated the balance of genetics and lifestyle influences, discovering that, while we cannot control our DNA, we may impact our aging process through good behaviors and decisions.

While aging is unavoidable, how we age is something we can actively control.

Chapter 2: Nutrition and Longevity

Your nutrition plays an important part in promoting longevity. Whole, plant-based diets, such as the Mediterranean, as well as anti-inflammatory diets, aid in protecting your cells. We found essential anti-aging nutrients, such as omega-3s, antioxidants, and polyphenols that promote health and combat inflammation.

A nutrient-dense, balanced diet can help you age gracefully from the inside out, and you can get started right now with a 7-day meal plan.

Chapter 3: Exercise and Movement for Life.

Physical activity is an essential component of aging properly. Movement promotes lifespan, whether through strength training to keep muscle, cardio to maintain heart health, or flexibility exercises to prevent injuries.

Regular exercise, customized to your fitness level, is critical to maintaining your strength, balance, and general health as you age.

Chapter 4: Mental Health and Aging

We investigated how mental health affects aging, including cognitive decline and emotional well-being. Mindfulness and meditation can help reduce stress and increase neuroplasticity, while emotional resilience is essential for dealing with the challenges of aging.

Cultivating a positive mentality, practicing mindfulness, and developing emotional resilience can help you safeguard your brain and live a happier, more purposeful life.

Chapter 5: Lifestyle Habits That Promote Longevity

Daily practices such as prioritizing sleep, intermittent fasting, and cultivating relationships all have a substantial impact on aging. Good sleep hygiene promotes cellular repair, whereas fasting and calorie restriction improve metabolic function. Strong social relationships also contribute to increased life expectancy.

Simple lifestyle practices like getting enough sleep, fasting, and maintaining meaningful connections can improve your health and longevity.

Chapter 6: Supplements and Cutting-Edge Anti-Aging Science

We looked at popular supplements like Vitamin D and resveratrol, as well as novel anti-aging techniques like fasting and cryotherapy. While promising, it's critical to stay current on evolving science.

Supplements and creative procedures may help you age better, but they should not substitute a healthy lifestyle.

Chapter 7: The Strength of Purpose and Positivity in Aging

A feeling of purpose is one of the most crucial aspects of having a long and fulfilled life. A positive mindset and emotional resilience can help you deal with the problems of aging while improving your mental and physical health.

Discovering and pursuing purpose at any age is essential for surviving, and maintaining a positive, adaptable mindset can increase your longevity and happiness.

Chapter 8: Real-Life Success Stories

Finally, we highlighted individuals who have used these ideas to achieve significant transformations. Their tales demonstrate that it is never too late to reinvent yourself, discover your purpose, and take steps toward a healthier, more vibrant existence.

The principles in this book are more than simply theory; they are instruments that can actually improve people's lives, as seen by these real-life examples.

Final Thoughts: Aging With Intention

As you move forward, keep in mind that aging should be celebrated rather than dreaded or resisted. With the knowledge and skills in this book, you may now make informed decisions that improve the quality and quantity of your life. By paying attention to your diet, physical health, mental well-being, and emotional resilience, you can age gracefully, vibrantly, and with a sense of purpose at every stage of your life.

You have the opportunity to shape your aging process—make it full of health, happiness, and meaning.

Start your journey to long-term health and vitality today.

You've just taken a deep dive into the science and tactics of aging gracefully, discovering that the secret to a long, vibrant life isn't just genetics, but also the daily decisions you make. Now it's time to put this knowledge into practice.

Do not wait for tomorrow or the ideal timing. The decisions you make today will shape your future health, energy, and happiness. **Every small step counts**, whether it's eating a more nutritious diet, starting a new fitness program, practicing mindfulness, or cultivating deeper relationships. When practiced consistently, these behaviors will change the way you age, allowing you to live not only longer but also better.

Begin simple:

• Try a new healthy dinner this week.

• Incorporate a brief daily stroll into your regimen.

• Do five minutes of mindfulness every morning.

• Connect with a friend or loved one to strengthen your social relationships.

These little, deliberate measures might result in significant shifts over time. **Your future self is waiting on you to get started today**—and the benefits are enormous: more energy, a sharper mind, stronger relationships, and a life full of purpose and happiness.

You have the tools. Now is the moment to take action. Begin using these tactics immediately to gain control of your aging process. Accept the path to a healthier, happier, and more fulfilling existence. **The best has yet to come!**

Final Thought: Healthy Aging is Within Your Control

Aging is unavoidable, but the way you age is mainly under your control. It's not about defying time but about embracing it and nurturing your body, mind, and soul via the decisions you make every day. The beauty of positive aging is that it does not necessitate major changes or perfection; it is about making tiny, consistent decisions in your daily life.

From the food you consume to the thoughts you have, the activities you engage in, and the relationships you nurture, these little, thoughtful actions add up over time to produce a life of health, longevity, and fulfillment. Every day is an opportunity to invest in your future well-being, to live with purpose, and to age gracefully but forcefully.

Remember, positive aging is achievable and within your reach. The journey begins with the decisions you make today.

9 798300 881429